35p

The Battle for Oblivion

———— * ————

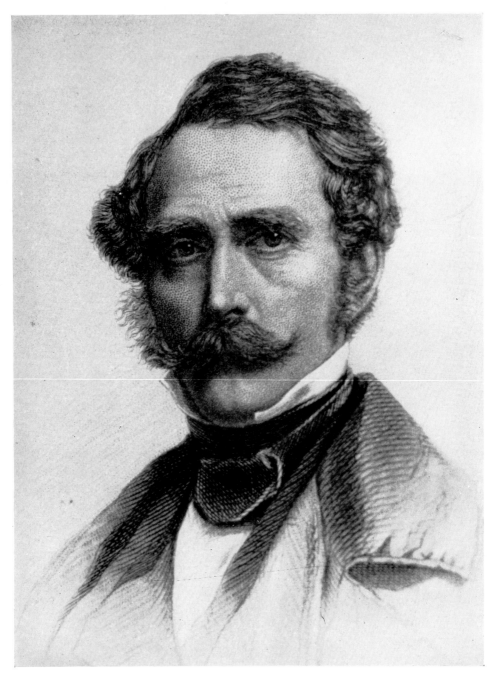

Portrait of William Morton

THE BATTLE
FOR
OBLIVION

The Discovery of Anaesthesia

by

BETTY MacQUITTY

With a Foreword by
CHRISTIAAN BARNARD

GEORGE G. HARRAP & CO. LTD
London · Toronto · Wellington · Sydney

First published in Great Britain 1969
by GEORGE G. HARRAP & Co. LTD
182 High Holborn, London, W.C. 1

SBN 245 59668 2

Composed in Intertype Period Old Style type and printed by
Cox & Wyman Ltd., London, Fakenham and Reading
Made in Great Britain

For thousands of years men had searched for relief from pain, but the anguished cries of humanity remained unanswered until a little more than a hundred years ago when an unknown American dentist, William Morton, discovered anaesthesia. Since that miraculous moment the terrifying agony of operations has been replaced by the painless sleep upon which modern surgery depends, but Morton, who suffered so much for his discovery, is still unknown to the millions who owe their lives to his work.

To WILLIAM MORTON
"Benefactor of Mankind"

FOREWORD

This is the story of a man who is still almost unknown even in medical circles, but without whose work modern surgery would be impossible. William Morton was a humble American dentist who discovered anaesthesia—one of the great advances made in medicine. It is told around his courageous fight against the prejudices of the medical profession of his day.

It seems incredible that only a little more than a hundred years ago all surgical operations were performed without anaesthesia. Patients were strapped and held down struggling on the operating table, and the agony of cutting for the stone or amputation of a limb was only reduced by the speed at which the surgeon worked. Legs were removed in as little as 25 seconds, and complicated operations were impossible. Today, thanks to Morton's discovery, the great surgeons of the world can carry out operations slowly and methodically, and the patient can be kept unconscious for many hours.

Great courage is necessary to be the first to try out new medical techniques, and every medical man will be able to appreciate the misgivings Morton felt when he took that enormous step into the unknown to demonstrate anaesthesia before the doctors and students assembled in the Ether Dome on October 16th, 1846.

The discovery of anaesthesia and Morton's struggle for recognition is moving and dramatic, and the medical profession is indebted to him for his great work. Betty MacQuitty is to be congratulated on producing a fitting memorial to a great man.

University of Cape Town

ACKNOWLEDGMENTS

I should like to acknowledge with gratitude all the facilities and kind help given to me by the Massachusetts General Hospital, Boston. My thanks are also due to the British Museum, the Council of the Royal College of Surgeons, the Royal College of Physicians, Mr W. R. Merrington, Curator to the University College Hospital Museum, Mr J. W. Barber-Lomax, Assistant-Director of the Wellcome Institute of the History of Medicine, the Boston City Library, the Boston Medical Library, the Harvard Medical Library, the Smithsonian Institution, and the members of their staff who gave me so much help in tracing sources and providing material; also the staff at the Farmington Library, who introduced me to the history of their beautiful town; *The Lancet* and *Illustrated London News* for the material quoted; Mr Henry Shaw and an old friend, Dr Lederman, and the Royal Marsden Hospital for their help.

Finally I am most grateful to that fine surgeon Professor Christiaan Barnard, who in spite of all his world commitments has found time to pay tribute to William Morton.

ILLUSTRATIONS

Plates in Half-tone

Line Drawings in the Text

1846

"WITH a meek, imploring look, and the startled air of a fawn, as her modest gaze meets the bold eyes fixed upon her, she is brought into the amphitheatre crowded with men anxious to see the shedding of her blood, and laid upon the table. With a knowledge and merciful regard to the intensity of the agony which she is to suffer, opiates and stimulants have been freely given her, which perhaps, at this stage, are again repeated. She is cheered by kind words, and the information that it will soon be over, and she freed for ever from what now afflicts her; she is enjoined to be calm, and to keep quiet and still and with assistance at hand to hold her struggling form, the operation is commenced.

"But of what avail are all her attempts at fortitude? At the first clear crisp cut of the scalpel, agonizing screams burst from her and with convulsive struggles she endeavours to leap from the table. But the force is nigh. Strong men throw themselves upon her and pinion her limbs. Shrieks upon shrieks make their horrible way into the stillness of the room, until the heart of the boldest sinks in his bosom like a lump of lead.

"At length it is finished, and, prostrated with pain, weak from her exertions, and bruised by the violence used, she is borne from the amphitheatre to her bed in the wards, to recover from the shock by slow degrees."[1]

This was the scene that William Morton set out to change.

[1] Nathan Rice, *Trials of a Public Benefactor* (New York, 1859).

CHAPTER

I

WILLIAM MORTON was born near Charlton, Massachusetts, on August 9th, 1819. His father's ancestors had come
from Scotland about the end of the seventeenth century with
the first thin stream of early immigrants. They were a hard-working, God-
fearing people, who had been hounded and persecuted by the established
Church in Britain. Forbidden to worship in their own way, they were
treated with the most appalling brutality. Forced off their land, informed
upon and harried by the King's men, they were constantly being brought
before magistrates and thrown into jail. Determined to work out their own
destiny, they sold up their possessions and, often embarking in the utmost
secrecy, prepared to brave the long, hard voyage. For some two months
they slept in filthy holds, and ate the meagre food they brought on board,
which ran out or went bad before the end of the journey. Subjected to
cholera, typhoid, and other deadly diseases, they survived the ordeal to
start again in the New World.

Robert Morton, one of the first of the family to arrive, started to
speculate and exchanged three shiploads of goods for several thousand
acres of land still unsettled in New Jersey. But the Mortons were too
simple in business and the land seemed to have been sold twice.
When the prosperous city of Elizabethtown grew up on their land it
was often suggested that the family should prosecute, but it would have
been too difficult and expensive to press the claim, and no attempt was
ever made.

Robert's son settled in a Quaker colony in Rhode Island, and when
their liberty again seemed in danger he was one of the first to answer the
call to arms to fight for their independence from the English. He was at
the famous battle of Bunker Hill, and his son fought alongside him too,
only to be killed tragically a few years after returning home to his wife and

family. Driving out in the chaise one day, the horse became unmanageable, and as he leapt out to seize the animal's head he fell on a scythe lying in the cart and soon bled to death. His small son James, then only a child of six years old, watched it happen and was deeply affected by the horror. His mother heroically worked the farm for him until he came of age, but when he married he gave it up and moved to where his wife lived near Charlton, Massachusetts. She came of a long line of prosperous farmers who had settled there at the beginning of the eighteenth century, and from her family he bought a farm of one hundred acres. Here, on August 9th, 1819, their son William Thomas Green Morton was born.

Already it was a United States of America vastly different from the country his ancestors had first set foot in. During that short time of one hundred years it had grown to a nation of nine million people, still less than every important country in Europe, but growing rapidly every year. Vast areas had been opened up and settled and the frontier pushed back. Yet it was still only an agricultural community that the child was born into, with few cities and no large industries, where people farmed or practised the simplest of trades. The Mortons lived in a plain, low, wooden weatherboard farmhouse, and surrounded by the same fields it stands there today —now nearly two hundred years old and almost forgotten—but still set solidly above the roaring traffic of the main trunk road below. When the Mortons lived there a brook near by was diverted from its course to supply the house with water, and in winter it became a skating-rink for the children.

The land was fertile, and each village had to exist on what food, fuel, and wool they could produce themselves. Their transactions were on a simple exchange basis, and when they took their wheat to the mill part of it went to pay for the milling; when their wool was cleaned and combed some paid for the processing. There were practically no foreign goods, and few comforts except the ones they made themselves. The winters there were long and bitter, and they had to grow enough in summer to carry them through. In autumn the dirt floors of the cellars were covered with barrels of salt pork and brine beef, with maple syrup, dried beans, and potatoes. As in all good New England households, the rafters in the Mortons' kitchen were hung with strings of dried apples, squashes, and pumpkins for the winter, with bunches of fennel and boneset for medicinal use. Their dresser was set out with bright burnished tins and quaint crockery. Their parlour was kept closed except for special occasions, and in the fashion of the day they hung its walls with paintings of hunting scenes and birds and fruit. The people were still sternly religious, and all in the Morton home was clean and plain, with a place for everything and everything in its place, for as is the place, so is the man, they said.

14

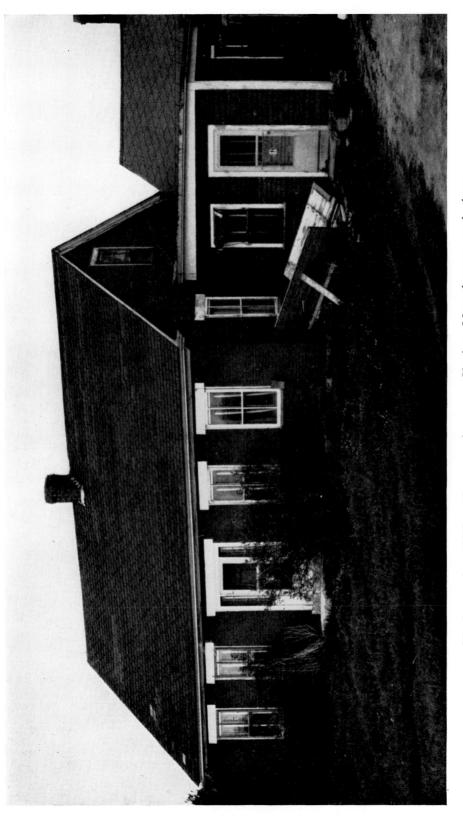

The house where William Morton was born, near Charlton, Massachusetts, stands almost unchanged today

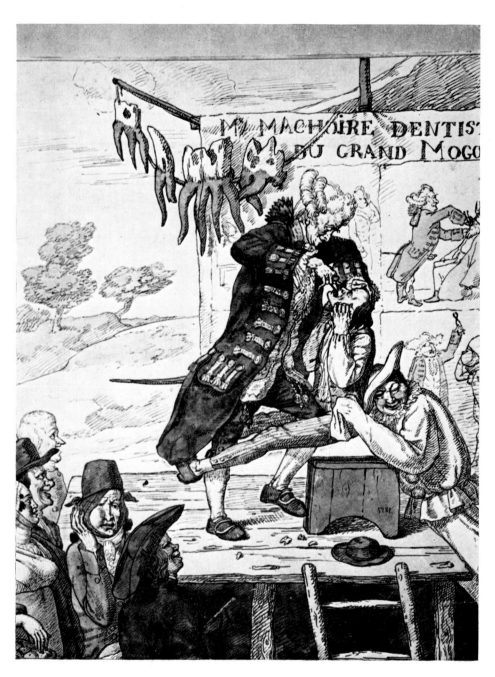

French cartoon of 1817 of a dentist

From just such backgrounds then as William Morton's, as out of chrysalises, burst the young virile sons of America determined to secure for themselves an honoured place in society. That education was the key to success was insisted upon by William's father. Denied a proper education himself through the tragic early death of his father, he was determined that his children should grasp what seemed unlimited opportunities for advancement, and his struggle to provide a good education dominated the boy's early life. William Morton was about eight years old when he started school, but it was only a tumbledown shack across fields and swamps, and it was almost impossible to get there in winter, the season when farming families could best spare time for education. James Morton wanted to sell up and move to a place where there was a proper school, but at first his wife was very much against it, for she was born there and her father had himself cleared the land and planted all the trees. Eventually James Morton got his way, the farm was sold, and the family moved into a house next door to the school in near-by Charlton. "I was twelve years old," says Morton, "when we moved to the little village where the church was; there I had a tolerable opportunity for attending school during the winter."[1] *

Even here the education was primitive, and James Morton decided that the only way to improve the standard of teaching for his children was to take an active part himself in the running of the school. He got appointed to the Board of Trustees and persuaded them to get a permanent master. He drove all the way to Brown University in Rhode Island to persuade a graduate from there to take the job, but unfortunately he did not last very long and the teaching lapsed into its bad old ways. Anyway, the pay was not much better than for a farm labourer, and sometimes a strip of land was planted with corn to pay the teacher's salary. They were expected to cope with pupils from the ages of six to as much as thirty, with up to eighty pupils cooped up in the one schoolroom, learning everything by rote, repeating it aloud after the teacher.

The young boy spent most of his time working on the farm, for with almost no mechanical help or hired labour the children had to work hard too. In spring they made the maple sugar, tapping the trees, catching the sap and evaporating it. Later in the year came the sheep-shearing, most of which the boys used to do, from the washing of the sheep to the carrying of the freshly cut fleeces to the mill, through its various stages of carding, hackling, and weaving, until it was ready for the tailor who travelled from house to house making up clothes for each family for the winter. In summer there was the mowing and haymaking, and the husking, paring, and drying of the apples for winter. As well as the farm jobs he learnt to skate, to fish and shoot, and lived the life of any other country boy.

* The notes relating to each chapter will be found at the end of the chapter.

15

Important too was his religious education, for he said later: "My mother has been a member of the Baptist Church ever since I can remember. It was her influence that educated me morally. The schoolhouse in the town was two miles from our residence, and through the woods and swamps. The church was further off but my mother always walked to church every Sabbath, rain or shine, and took me with her."[2]

William Morton had always wanted to learn medicine, and when he used to dose his friends with a battery of elder-tree pills they nicknamed him "The Doctor". But he had to be forbidden such unorthodox practices after he had nearly killed his little sister by pouring down her throat some dreadful concoction of his own as she lay asleep in her cradle. When he was about thirteen William was sent to an Academy in Oxford, a small town near by. Here he stayed with the family of Dr Pierce, an old friend of his mother's and a physician with quite a local reputation. His stay with Dr Pierce spurred him on in his ambition, and his father urged him, too, saying "to be a doctor was to be somebody and to have a respected place in the community". There the boy spent hours poring over the medical books, but the doctor must have got tired of the boy's rhapsodies on the pleasures of the medical profession, for he is said to have retorted, "Young man, you hardly know what you talk about and how hard I have to work."[3]

William Morton had been at the Oxford Academy for only just over a year when one of the boys falsely accused him of disobeying some school rule. The teacher refused to believe Morton's statement that he was innocent and insisted that he must make a full confession. Still the boy stuck to his story that he had done nothing wrong. He must have known that if he held out against the teacher he would be very heavily punished, but in spite of all attempts to make him confess he still denied the accusation. Later in life he was to show the same stubborn determination to stick to the truth and to persist, also in the face of great opposition, in the mistaken belief that justice must eventually prevail. His refusal to back down was followed by an "ill-judged and outrageous punishment", which led to his leaving school and returning home. There is no mention of what the punishment was, but the education of children in America at that time was very severe, with the cat-o'-nine-tails and whipping-posts still there to drive out the devil from them. His punishment was so harsh that his health was ruined, and according to his family for many months he was unfit for thought or action.

While recuperating William helped his father in the village store he had bought. There he smelt "the bolted cloth, fish, coffee and snuff" and listened to "the sound of the molasses keg dripping rhythmically".[4] He read a lot and explored the hills and woods, from where he could see the white buildings of the Town Meeting House, the Congregational and

16

Universalist churches with their prim spires, the old Burying Ground, and the little weather-board houses clustering around.

After a summer at home the boy was sent to an Academy in Northfield, far away in the hills near the State border and a long six-hour coach journey from home. He was a sensitive boy and was so homesick there that eventually his father took him away and put him nearer home at the Leicester Academy. These academies had sprung up everywhere to cope with the demand for a better education, for families like the Mortons had money to spare now and were eager for a more gentlemanly education for their sons. The boy spent nearly two years at Leicester, and was described by his classmates as indefatigable in his efforts to acquire information on all subjects. While his companions played he was supposed to have spent his time searching the hills for mineral specimens. He was very happy there, and would have remained to finish his education but for the sudden change in his father's situation.

Until now it had been boom time in America, and the Mortons had been carried forward on the tide of prosperity with all the rest. James Morton had broken away from the land and from farming as his ancestors had done, ran the village store, and launched out into other business ventures. Everything was on the up and up, and prices soared higher and higher. Land changed hands many times, and in Chicago land which at the beginning of the century had been sold for $1.25 an acre, by 1832 went for $100 and by 1834 made $3500. Eventually the situation got completely out of hand and prices impossible. To stop them rocketing further the Government suddenly insisted that all land must be paid for in gold or silver. Immediately there was panic throughout the country. Banks and businesses could not meet the tremendous demand for coin and everywhere went bankrupt, until even the central Government itself could no longer pay its debts. Senator Benton of Missouri described the situation: "The goods are worn out, the paper money has returned to the place whence it came; the operation is over, and nothing remains to the transactions but the 170 million in debt. . . . The whole of these banks have failed once, and most of them twice, in two years. . . ." America was in a desperate way, and when in 1842 an envoy of the Government approached the Rothschilds of Paris to ask for a loan he was told: "You may tell your government that you have seen the man who is at the head of the finances of Europe and that he has told you that they cannot borrow a dollar, not a dollar."

The bubble of boom and good fortune had finally burst, and in a crisis of such magnitude no one in America remained untouched by its frightful consequences. James Morton had gone into a mercantile co-partnership and lost all his money. He had to sell up everything and to take his son away from school, and Morton says: "I was there (at Leicester Academy) when the news of the failure of my father—utterly unexpected by his family—reached me and ended my school education. My father lost all his property, our family were scattered and for several years had no home together."[5]

So, at the age of seventeen, William was forced to leave school to try to earn his own living. Jobs were not easy to come by, but luckily through friends of the family he managed to get a position in Boston in the printing firm of James B. Dow. Dow was the editor of the *Christian Witness*, and he and Mrs Dow took a great personal interest in the boy. But Boston was a very different place from the village that Morton had known. It was an important seaport and trading town, handling more than a thousand foreign ships each year. Looking like an old English seafaring town, it was full of little shops of every sort—tailors, wig-makers, chandlers, ship-suppliers, all crowded together beside trading houses and banks. Thronged with merchants and sailors, its narrow, winding cobbled streets led down to wharves lined with ships busily unloading immigrants and foreign goods in exchange for American agricultural products. By day it was bright and bustling, full of high morality and decent trade, but at night its badly lit streets became the haunt of drunken sailors.

To the young country boy it seemed a marvellous and exciting place, full of interesting people and opportunities to learn. Here he first met Mrs Sarah Hale, the celebrated editor of various ladies' magazines and the author of the famous nursery rhyme "Mary had a little lamb, Its fleece as white as snow". She says: "I knew Willie Morton as a clerk in the publication office of my magazine. . . . His early training must have had a salutary influence in keeping him from the evil temptations so often destructive of those left early to self-guidance."[6] She describes him as already dedicated: "Morton did not think merely about a living as most would; it was, to the subject of our notice, not a mere living but a living to some purpose of improvement and essential advancement for the future." Mrs Hale's ladies' magazines were full of such high moralizing, for Massachusetts was still a Puritan stronghold.

Morton had not entirely given up the idea of becoming a doctor, and he searched desperately for some way of making enough money to pay for his medical training: "enterprising and intelligent," Mrs Hale says, "he sought in various places to establish himself in business." But it was difficult to make money in those hard times, and he had no more idea of business and its sharp practices than his father. No judge when it came to choosing suitable business partners, and "duped by designing men" older and shrewder and better versed in business, his mercantile career soon ended in disaster. Disappointed, he fled back home to Charlton.

18

NOTES TO CHAPTER I

1. A letter from Morton quoted by Mrs Sarah J. Hale in *Godey's Lady's Book,* 1853.
2. *Ibid.*
3. Nathan Rice, *Trials of a Public Benefactor* (New York, 1859). This book is largely Morton's own story, for the material in it, including a vast number of letters and documents, was supplied by Morton. In fact Rice complained after it was printed that the title and much of the book was written by Morton himself.
4. Sarah J. Hale, *op. cit.*
5. *Ibid.*
6. *Ibid.*

II

MORTON was now a young man of twenty-one, tall and handsome, with fine features and a good bearing. He dressed carefully, and although he had little money to spend on clothes he always managed to look neat and presentable. Back home again in Charlton, he had to admit that he had no hope now of finding enough money for medical studies, and decided that the next best thing would be to become a dentist instead. Up to that time doctors had extracted teeth, but also, hanging about fairgrounds and such public places, were men who called themselves dentists. But few of them were skilled or educated men, for dentists needed no qualifications, no degrees, and no licence to practise, and began simply as apprentices, picking up what little knowledge they could as they went along. Dr Chapin A. Harris, who did so much to put dental surgery on a proper footing in America, said: "The calling of the dentist has been resorted to by the ignorant and illiterate, and I am sorry to say in too many instances by unprincipled individuals."[1] Happy to take money off anyone gullible enough to employ them, a writer describes one of them in action: "Slowly, and with due regard to the anxious patient . . . shown by brandishing the forceps before his eyes—the quack then proceeds to seize the offending member. With the delicacy of a blacksmith, and the skill of a hod-carrier, the practitioner immediately twists the crown of the tooth from the roots, and leaving the fangs as before embedded in the jaw, advises the sufferer to return to his domicile, exercise his patience, and obtain what relief he can, not forgetting at the same time to remind him of the fee demanded for his valuable services."[2]

But about this time steps were beginning to be taken to exercise some sort of control over dentists, and in 1840 the first college, the Baltimore College of Dental Surgery, was opened and the American Society of Dental Surgeons formed. Morton went to see Dr Horace Hayden, Presi-

20

dent of the Society and a professor at the new college, and became one of his first students. Mrs Hale mentions a legacy which enabled him to begin his studies and that "he divided his time between the counter and the schoolroom, going from one to the other and saving from his earnings as a clerk to pay the expenses of his tuition as a pupil".[3] Morton probably also worked as a dental apprentice.

In 1842 at the age of twenty-three Morton set up practice near Hartford, Connecticut. He already knew another dentist, Horace Wells, who practised in Hartford itself. Wells was a clever and ambitious man and had already written a manual on dentistry. Morton learnt a great deal about the profession from him, and, indeed, may have worked as an apprentice to Wells before setting up in Farmington and Cheshire, two townships not far from Wells's own practice.

Wells was nearly two years older than Morton. He was an exuberant character with red hair and bright-blue eyes, a round, soft face, and bushy side-whiskers, and was always bubbling over with some bright scheme for making a fortune. Morton was ambitious too, and they both had high hopes for the future. Wells had just invented a new type of dental solder for attaching artificial teeth to plates, which was non-corrosive and was supposed to prevent the galvanic action that produced an unsightly black line around the margin of the teeth and gave off an unpleasant taste and smell. The two of them decided to set up as partners to exploit the invention, and with the one thousand dollars Morton had borrowed from an old lady they went off to Boston to put up their plate outside 19 Tremont Row in the heart of the city. In this vast and bustling metropolis they felt sure that patients would soon come flocking into their surgery to try out their new invention.

Wells took out a patent for his new solder, and they applied to Dr Charles Jackson for a certificate of approval. Jackson was a very eminent Boston chemist, and as soon as they got his certificate that the solder was effective and not harmful they advertised extensively in newspapers and quoted Jackson on its chemical properties. Dentists were still not much better than hucksters peddling their wares, and advertising was not only not forbidden, but was recognized as normal practice. Baits of all kinds were offered to potential patients, and Morton and Wells themselves guaranteed patients their money back if after one year they were not satisfied with the new treatment. The young partners sat back then to wait for the patients to roll in. But in spite of all their efforts to promote their practice—and the cut prices they offered—they had little business, for their new treatment depended upon the removal of the teeth, stumps perhaps left in by other incompetent dentists, and this was so painful that, although a lot of patients climbed the stairs to their surgery, most of them scuttled down again very quickly.

When Wells saw that he was not going to make a fortune after all, he decided to withdraw from the partnership and go back to his old practice in Hartford. He was an impetuous man, clever and ingenious, always seizing eagerly on new ideas and methods, but never working at them long enough to make a success. He spent his whole life jumping from one stunt to another, always bursting with enthusiasm about the money which he was going to make, but never remaining long enough to reap the rewards. Now, after only a short time in partnership with Morton, he decided to quit, to pack up and go back to Hartford. In a letter dated November 22nd, 1843, he gave notice to Morton of his intention to withdraw:

> We can both of us see at a glance that it is madness for us to go ahead under present circumstances, for the reason that our receipts will barely pay the cost of materials used, even if we had ever so much work at the prices you have taken those jobs now on hand. . . . I am satisfied in my own mind that our enterprise will be a total failure. So, let us give it up and jog along here at home as usual; in case you do not give up the enterprise, I of course am ready and do give you notice that I wish to get out of it as soon as our agreement will permit. I wish you to understand that I have not the least fault to find with you; I have the utmost confidence in you as a gentleman, and one who will ever aim to act your part well in accordance with the strictest honour and integrity; we have both exerted ourselves to the utmost, and I believe that our ill-success cannot be attributed to either of us so far as 'goaheaditiveness' is concerned.[4]

One of their last joint enterprises was the exhibition in 1844 of a case of dental instruments, for which they received a diploma from the Massachusetts Mechanical Association, and the final notice of dissolution appeared in the *Boston Daily Atlas* of October 24th, 1844.

But if Wells gave up, Morton was certainly not ready to do so. When Wells went back to Hartford he struggled desperately on in Boston, and here was the vital difference between the two men. While Wells always threw in his hand if the enterprise was not an immediate success, Morton clung on tenaciously, prepared to work carefully and methodically to improve the idea until he had turned failure into success. And it was this tremendous capacity for hard work and experimentation which enabled Morton to triumph and the lack of which destined Wells for failure.

But for Morton it meant desperately hard work to keep going. He slept on a couch in his surgery and worked all hours of the day there, trying always to appear neat and well groomed. At first he was too poor to own all his instruments, and for complicated cases he had to borrow. Slowly, and with a great deal of hard and grinding work, he built up a modest practice. But still the most difficult problem was how to improve his knowledge of the subject. There were no good textbooks, and other dentists refused to give him any help, for each dentist had his own methods, his own jealously guarded secrets, and his reputation and his income de-

22

pended on keeping these to himself. Carefully Morton began to try to work out the best methods for himself by trial and error. He also paid five hundred dollars for the knowledge and trade secrets of Dr Nathan C. Keep, Vice-President of the American Society of Dental Surgeons. For this money Keep was willing to throw open the doors of his laboratory and to give Morton the benefit of his experience. Keep also gave him a testimonial describing Morton as "a very enterprising dentist—his mind ever active and seeking for improvement". "I have taken great pleasure in exchanging professional thoughts with him," said Keep, "and am desirous of promoting his honourable intentions."[5]

Armed with Keep's testimonial, Morton set about building up a good practice. Nothing was too much trouble for him, and everything, even the most difficult cases, he tackled with the most painstaking care. He had read about a French dentist who a century before had made a gold crown to cover a decayed tooth of the King's mistress, after which replacement of teeth became the work of goldsmiths—then ivory workers when dental plates with the teeth included were carved out of ivory. Later on hippopotamus and then human teeth were preferred and set into plates. A fine haul of teeth was made from the bodies of soldiers strewn over the battlefield at Waterloo, and crates of them were imported into England to be used in dental plates, but there was such an outcry that people were put off using them.

Now in the United States properly qualified dentists began to crown teeth and provide plates. Morton was a good technician and tried his hand at this sort of work. He was soon so successful that he was making plates not only for his own patients, but for other dentists as well. For a young man who had a hare-lip, cleft palate, deficient palatine arch and nasal septum, he made a gold plate on which were the three deficient front teeth. He adjusted it so accurately that the deformity was much less obvious, and eventually the young man was able to talk almost normally. His work on these cases was commended by doctors and elocutionists. He even made a false nose for a woman who had lost hers: "Having taken an accurate mould from a dwarf in the city who was noted for the beauty and symmetry of her nasal protuberance, an exact copy was made by Dr Morton in plantina and enamelled. This, coloured as nearly to life as art could make it, was attached to her spectacles. With this accessory appendage well adjusted, and a piece of court plaster placed as a beauty spot upon her forehead to act as a foil and attract the attention of those who saw her, the defect was hardly to be noticed."[6]

From all this dental work Morton began gradually to make a profit, and within a year he was able to pay back the thousand dollars he had borrowed. The income from his practice rose to around twenty thousand dollars a year, and he got so many orders for making false teeth that he opened a factory. A newspaper of the day described it:

Our curiosity had been awakened by hearing that a show-case, destined for the London Exhibition, of which we spoke a fortnight since, was to contain nearly one hundred thousand false teeth! And having visited nearly every description of 'mill' in various quarters of the globe, we had curiosity to examine a Tooth Mill! Our curiosity was gratified in the most obliging manner and we, kind reader, will now pass with you through his (Morton's) large establishment. . . .

Entering, we first examine a steam engine, throbbing away like a fettered giant, yet obedient as a child to its vigilant director. He has but to move a finger, and his iron slave, still pursuing its labour, pumps water, blows the fire, or propels supplementary mechanical devices, of which we shall hereafter speak.

Now we enter the 'Mill' proper, where the stones revolve with fearful velocity, and send forth a delicate flour. Taste it not, unless you wish to have your teeth set on edge, for it is pulverised stone; ay, and that of the hardest kind, as you may see by examining one of the lumps in yonder pile. Let us take one of those, and have it put through by the workmen.

The quarry whence this obdurate mass of quartz and spar comes is in New Jersey, whence tons are brought to the factory by iron horse. Once in this establishment, it is broken into small pieces, and the best bits are culled with care.

They go into the mill, whose hard quartz stones revolve, with almost electrical swiftness. "Munch, munch, munch", as said the chestnut-eating dame in *Macbeth*. Out it comes, at last, in a white, pure-looking powder, which resembles pulverised pearls, sprinkled with diamond dust.[7]

The article goes on to describe the kneading, moulding, firing, and finally the enamelling of the teeth and plates. From all this and from his growing practice Morton began to make a handsome profit. He had weathered the initial difficulties of establishing himself in the profession, and at last for him the tide began to turn.

NOTES TO CHAPTER II

1. Chapin A. Harris, *Address to American Society of Dental Surgeons*.
2. Nathan Rice, *Trials of a Public Benefactor*.
3. Sarah J. Hale, *Godey's Lady's Book*.
4. Nathan Rice, *op. cit.* (Material supplied by Morton.)
5. *Ibid.*
6. *Ibid.*
7. *Ibid.*

CHAPTER

III

WHEN Morton first started as a dentist in 1842 he had set up practice in Farmington, Connecticut, and it was here shortly afterwards that he met Elizabeth Whitman, a niece of the old lady who had lent him the thousand dollars to go to Boston to set up practice with Wells. Farmington was a typical little New England settlement about nine miles from Hartford. It survives there today—a suburb of Hartford now—but still standing in all its pristine glory, its beautiful weather-board houses clustering round the shining white wooden Congregational church. With its tall elegant spire it is the third and biggest church to be built there, and Samuel Whitman, one of Elizabeth's ancestors, was its first pastor. She writes: "Two of my Whitman ancestors, father and son, graduated at Harvard, one in 1668 and the other in 1696. The son settled in Farmington as one of the earliest ministers",[1] and for forty-five years preached the Gospel to the people of Farmington. His successors became farmers and landowners in and around the town, and when Morton met Elizabeth the Whitman family was wealthy and wielded considerable influence in the district.

Morton was twenty-three and Elizabeth just sixteen when they first met at a dance held at the Elm Tree Inn, a beautiful white wooden building dating from 1638, with green shutters and shaded by the large elm-trees brought from a swamp. Elizabeth Whitman was small and delicate, with a pale beautiful face and lovely dark eyes. When Morton saw her there at the dance he fell in love with her at first sight, for her voice, her figure, her movements, everything about her, aroused his keen admiration. "I learned later on," she says, "that from the first day he saw me he had determined to marry me if he could, and after his death I found in an old diary of that year an entry written just after my first meeting with him,

25

where he expressed his intention of making me his wife, and even noted the gown and hood I wore."[2]

After the dance Elizabeth Whitman asked Morton to call, but her parents were very annoyed at such a low character as a dentist paying court to their daughter. As she says: "I being a young girl of 17, just out of Miss Porter's school at Farmington, Connecticut, where my father lived. For a year before Dr Morton had paid me attentions which were not well received by my family, he being regarded as a poor young man with an undesirable profession. I thought him very handsome, however, and he was very much in love with me, coming regularly from Boston to visit me."[3]

Morton knew that the Whitman family considered him a most unsuitable suitor for their daughter's hand and set about trying to improve himself and to earn enough money to overcome their opposition. His struggle to make money was difficult enough, but becoming a respected member of society appeared almost impossible. He grew moustaches, which he thought made him look older and more dignified. He became a member of their Congregational church, very much the establishment Church in New England. But still the family refused to consider having a dentist as a prospective son-in-law, for dentists were regarded as disreputable characters not generally received in polite society. There were long family arguments. Elizabeth insisted she would marry no one else. Her father remained adamant. But her aunt supported the young people's cause and pointed out that the young man was ambitious and would soon make his way in the world.

Eventually, when Elizabeth still held out, the Whitmans agreed to accept him as a son-in-law, but only provided he agreed to become a doctor instead. They felt a doctor might just possibly be acceptable in the family, for as Morton's father had continually told him, "to be a doctor is to be somebody and to have a respected place in the community". Morton, of course, could not have been happier about the decision, for not only was he to marry the girl he loved, but he would also now fulfil his lifelong ambition to become a doctor.

Morton enrolled as a medical student in March 1844, carrying on his work as a dentist and studying medicine at the same time. And in May of that year the couple were married. The ceremony was performed by Noah Porter, who was for so many years pastor of the Congregational church, the father of Sarah Porter, headmistress of Elizabeth's old school, the now famous Miss Porter's School in Farmington. The marriage took place in the "immaculate, flower-draped parlour" of the Whitmans' house. Elizabeth's mother wrote describing it to her son in Boston:

It has been a very busy and interesting time with me and I suppose you have got the bridegroom and bride with you in Boston. The wedding passed off very pleasantly and I believe much to the satisfaction of all present. Most all of the young ladies and gentlemen of your acquaintance were here. It was truly delightful to see so much youth and beauty on such an occasion. W. and E. appeared very dignified and composed during the ceremony. They were both dressed very handsomely for the occasion. You never saw E. look more sweetly. She wore a pretty white muslin dress and long flowing white veil.

The young ladies were all dressed very handsomely. Many of them had new dresses for the occasion. There was much excitement and preparation with them for a few days previous and *all* seemed to take an interest. Charlie Norton and many of the little girls brought a profusion of beautiful flowers on the morning of the day and our friends cheerfully supplied us with silver cake baskets, china plates, glasses and shades, and coloured lamps.

We had an abundance of cake and a large tub of lemonade. We had two coloured men dressed in white coats and long white aprons to serve and three women to superintend other matters.

The happy pair were pronounced by some to make decidedly the best appearance of any in the party. The young gents prepared a few tunes for the occasion, and after the lights were out for the night gave the married pair a pleasant serenade.

Perhaps they sang some of the popular songs of that time, like *Jim Crow*, *Pretty Polly Perkins of Paddington Green*, *Limerick Races*, or *Home Sweet Home*, or even the *Anacreontic Song*, a drinking song which was later to become America's national anthem, the *Star-Spangled Banner*.

So at the age of eighteen Elizabeth became Mrs William Morton and "left the fine old homestead we lived in, quite an historical mansion it was from where John C. Calhoun (who became Vice-President of the United States) often visited my father's family".[4] Roads in America were still in a deplorable state and stagecoaches old and rickety, and the couple travelled more comfortably by water, down the canal from Farmington to New Haven, and from there by packet steamer to Boston.

After the small village of Farmington, Boston must have seemed an enormous city indeed to the young bride. She knew of Morton's ambitions, but even she must have been surprised at how hard her husband worked and with what devotion to the subject. Her husband, she said, "was one of those tremendously earnest men who believe they have a high destiny to fulfil. . . . Never shall I forget my sensation as a young bride at sleeping in a room where a tall, gaunt skeleton stood in a big box near the head of the bed. . . . During our early married life while he was making himself one of the most skilful dentists in Boston and carrying on an enormous business, he found time in addition to pursue his studies at Harvard Medical School in order to take up medicine. Every morning he rose between four and five to get time for what he called his *serious work*."[5]

27

Morton's wedding gave fresh stimulus to his ambitions. Here he was married at last to the girl he loved so dearly, well on the road to fulfilling his life's ambition to be a doctor, and although it was hard work running his practice and carrying on his medical studies, nothing now stood in his way. Everything Morton set out to achieve he did with immense thoroughness and concentration, and when he began his medical studies at Harvard he enrolled as a student of Dr Jackson's and also went with his wife to board with him as well. Jackson was the eminent chemist to whom he and Wells had applied for a certificate of approval for their new solder. He was a qualified doctor, a noted geologist, and a professor at Harvard, and in time became State geologist for Maine, Rhode Island, and New Hampshire, and Master of the State mint. After graduating from Harvard he had studied in Paris and Europe, and now at the age of thirty-nine was known in Europe as well as in the United States.

At his home up on Beacon Hill in Boston Jackson had set up a large and well-equipped laboratory, and Morton had the use of this and of Jackson's excellent scientific library. By boarding with him Morton was also able to talk to Jackson at meal-times and so on, and found his advice on medical and scientific matters most useful. But Morton had to be careful, for Jackson was a very difficult person and was especially scathing to juniors. He was an arrogant man who could not stand his judgement being questioned, or being crossed or thwarted in any way. Morton took care to be suitably deferential to him, and managed to get along pretty well most of the time.

Testimonials were considered essential for professional men at that time, and Morton received one from Jackson which read:

Mr W. T. G. Morton, dentist, entered his name with me as a student of medicine, 20 March 1844 and attended practical anatomy in the Massachusetts Medical College during the winter of that year; where he dissected with diligence and zeal and paid special attention to the anatomy of the head and throat—parts of the human anatomy particularly important to the surgeon-dentist.

He also studied Bell's and other standard works on anatomy and attended the lectures of Dr Warren, Dr Hayward and other professors.

I would recommend him as a suitable person for admission as a dental surgeon. He is a skilful operator in dentistry, both in the surgical and mechanical departments, and has studied the chemical properties of the ingredients required for the manufacture of artificial teeth.[6]

Morton matriculated on November 6th, 1844, and started his medical studies at Harvard Medical School, then on Mason Street, in the heart of Boston. He listened with awe to all the great figures there: John Collins Warren, the great American surgeon who had been trained in London and Paris and who was the first in America to operate for a strangulated hernia; George Hayward, his assistant; Channing, the Dean of the Harvard Medical School, who taught midwifery and had a constant stream of good stories; and Jacob Bigelow, a popular man with a cultivated taste who always taught him sympathetically and intelligently. He was also taught chemistry by John White Webster (later to come to a bad end when he murdered Professor George Parkman), a "short, thick set man . . . with his restless, ever watchful eyes partially concealed by gold spectacles—one moment explaining some point or elucidating some theory; at the next dashing, in an apparently reckless and careless manner, among his curiously shaped jars and various apparatus and concealed troughs, to establish the fact in the performance of the experiment."[7]

As part of his studies Morton also had to spend time in the dissecting room:

> That golgotha whose secrets are so faithfully kept from the prying world. The long low room, dimly lighted from above; the rows of dark red wooden tables, the students laughing about in their red woollen shirts, knit caps and india-rubber sleeves; some smoking cigars, or short clay pipes, chatting or cracking jokes; other busily engaged in their work over some unsightly relic of humanity; the nauseating odour which pervaded the air, in no wise favourably neutralized by the clouds of tobacco smoke; the blood dripping to the floor from many a divided vein; the bits of flesh, hair, and bones, scattered at random over the dirty floor; the broken coffins piled in the corners; and the sole ornaments, some grinning skeletons [that had he not been so keen to learn he would have gladly escaped].[8]

While doing all this studying Morton had to keep his dental work going as well. His practice was now a great success, and he employed several apprentices, but supervised all the work himself. He was making good money, and although it was all very hard work, his life was immensely satisfying. His speciality was replacing and crowning teeth, and he had invented a lute with which crowns of teeth could be attached. But here again he was brought up against the insuperable problem that to fix this on properly the patient had to suffer considerable, and usually unbearable, pain. It shows what an enormous debt humanity owes to Morton that today it is difficult to imagine the terrible pain suffered when teeth are extracted without anaesthetics. In fact, pulling teeth has always been a most effective form of torture. St Apollonia and Blasius the Blessed were tied to pillars while their teeth were extracted to persuade them to renounce Christianity, and King John used to pull out teeth as a means of extortion. When a wealthy citizen of Bristol refused to give the ten thousand ducats that the King demanded, the tyrant had him brought to the palace. With his own royal hands he extracted one tooth every day for a week, until the poor man could endure it no longer and paid up.

It was this intolerable pain that Morton wanted to save his patients, and

29

it was to this that he now devoted so much of his time. He read everything he could about pain-killers. He tried everything he had ever heard of: brandy, champagne, and other alcohols (in such large doses that the patient was completely intoxicated but unfortunately still conscious of the pain); opium, and laudanum in doses of one hundred to three hundred drops. One entry in his notebook reads:

> Mrs S. to have the whole of teeth in both jaws extracted. Commenced giving opiates about noon. Gave first one hundred and fifty drops of laudanum. Twenty minutes later, gave one hundred and fifty additional. Waited ten minutes and gave one hundred drops more. Gave two hundred drops more with intervals of five minutes. Whole amount given, five hundred drops in forty five minutes. At the expiration of this, she was sleepy, but able to walk to the chair. Immediately on extraction of the first tooth, she vomited. She continued in this way for one hour, during which time the rest of the teeth were extracted. She was conscious, but insensible to considerable degree. On returning home, she continued to vomit at intervals during the afternoon.[9]

Morton also tried opium in masses of ten or twelve grains, but although all made the patients sick and ill, none of them effectively alleviated the pain. Morton's search was an ancient problem, for throughout the ages men had sought a way to relieve pain. In primitive societies the witch-doctor tries to cast out the demon. From the early days of Christianity the laying on of hands or the touching by kings was supposed to effect a cure. The Egyptians believed that the root of mandragora was the gift to them of Ra, their sun-god, and that it took away pain, and the Greeks believed that Aphrodite cast herself into a bed of lettuce and mandragora to relieve her grief at the death of Adonis. St Benedict was supposed to have put the Emperor Henry II to sleep on a mandragora pillow before amputating his leg. The Egyptians used poppies too, and one of their princes found relief from sleeping on a bed of them. Raw opium was popular with the Chinese, and Indian hemp or hashish had an equally old history. But the results from all these so-called pain-killers were never consistent and the outcome always incalculable. The principal difficulty was to separate the drug from the poison, and an overdose meant certain death. In fact, the dangers were considered too great to justify their use, and the law imposed heavy penalties on those who tried to administer them. In the seventeenth century Bailly, a barber-surgeon of Troyes, put one of his patients to sleep with a herbal syrup before an operation, and all the other doctors rose in indignation. Gui Patin, a doctor and renowned man of letters attached to the University of Paris, addressed a protest to the medical faculty of Troyes: "If Bailly really uses narcotic plants in this way, you had better take him soundly to task. Herbal poisons have worked mischief in more skilful hands than his. See to it that these practices are not allowed, and do not let him go unpunished. The impudent barber should not be able to

30

boast of having done such things with impunity." Bailly had to pay a very heavy fine, and the use of herbal remedies to stupefy patients before operations was forbidden.

Morton studied all these drugs, and was prepared to try anything to help his patients, even mesmerism. The man who first propounded its extraordinary theories, Anton Mesmer, had begun as a student of divinity and law, but went on to take a degree in medicine. He lived in the eighteenth century, when natural laws were being discovered which appeared to govern the world instead of those of God, and he believed that the sun, moon, and stars influenced "all organized bodies by means of a mobile fluid, which pervades the whole universe and draws all things together in mutual intercourse and harmony."[10] At first he maintained that this force was electricity, then magnetism, and that it was only necessary for him to place his two magnets in contact with the patient's body and they would immediately feel better, for the healing fluid flowed through their body and restored it to harmony with the universe. He was thrown out of Vienna for his practices, but moved to Paris and set himself up there as a prophet of his new philosophy. He began to collect disciples and proclaimed: "I am the one through whom the universal healing fluid becomes effective. These cosmic energies which can heal every disease, mitigate every pain, radiate from my hands and from my words."[11]

So many patients flooded into his house in Montmartre—the whole of the Paris Court, Marie Antoinette herself, and Lafayette—that it was soon impossible to treat them all individually, and he then began charging various objects. At first he ranged great numbers of sick people round a big wooden tub filled with bottles of water he was supposed to have magnetized, connecting them to it by cords and bars. The patients received their magnetism through these and from the wand and touch of the magnetizer. The sounds of a piano or some compelling voice was also supposed to diffuse the magnetism in the air, and the patients had to sit there for an hour so that their bodies could be charged. Often they suffered convulsions, and the performance was so popular that Parisians had to reserve a place many days in advance. The wealthy and aristocratic of France would invite their friends to a seat there, and the show was as good as having a box at the Comédie. Everyone was so impressed with Mesmer's healing powers that when Lafayette went to America he told Washington that besides bringing munitions to help the United States in their fight for freedom from the British, he also brought the most wonderful gift of mesmerism, "a marvellous weapon against illness and pain".

When the demand increased still further and his munificent consulting rooms in the Place Vendôme were crowded out Mesmer had to treat smaller tubs to be sold for home use. He magnetized bowls in which the thousands of sick could wash away their pains, mirrors before which the patients filed to look at their image and to receive the magnetic current

31

which would make them well, and he even sold musical instruments, the notes of which silenced the pain. Still he could not satisfy the demand, and he transferred his powers to the open country: gardens, parks, shrubs, even whole forests, were magnetized. To be cured the sick had merely to tie themselves with ropes to the trees which Mesmer had charged with the fluid. In the Rue Bondi, day after day, hundreds of people flocked to an oak-tree there to be relieved of their pain.

The French believed Mesmer was their most precious possession, and were very worried about what would happen when he died. Would his power die with him, and would the power of the tubs and trees and bowls then evaporate? The State offered to build an institute for him to work in and to give him a pension of forty thousand *livres* if only he would pass on his powers to certain persons nominated by it. Mesmer was prepared to agree providing he had official scientific recognition of his discovery, something so far he had been unable to secure. Some doctors and scientists supported him, but most were openly contemptuous. "It is impossible to conceive the sensation which Mesmer's experiments created in Paris," said Baron Dupotet. "No theological controversy in the earlier ages of the Church was ever conducted with greater bitterness."[12]

Louis XVI intervened and persuaded the Academy of Sciences to hold an inquiry into the effects of Mesmer's animal magnetism. The committee contained some of the most famous men of the day: Dr Guillotin, who was so concerned to see that prisoners were killed quickly and humanely that he invented the gruesome device which now bears his name; Benjamin Franklin, the discoverer of the lightning conductor; the famous chemist Lavoisier; and other distinguished members.

In their report they tried to be tactful, but concluded that although Mesmer's treatment did involve something they could not explain, they were unable to give it their approval. Mortified, Mesmer announced that he was going to leave Paris. The Queen was in despair. Maurepas, the Minister of State, offered him every conceivable honour and a large sum of money in compensation, but Mesmer remained unmoved. To mollify him his supporters set up the Société Harmonique to raise money for him to have his own Academy in opposition to the official Academy of Sciences. In return Mesmer was to place at the Society's disposal a number of mesmerized objects and to instruct the members in his methods. To finance this scheme the Society issued shares of one hundred *louis* each. It was declared an impossible fee, but even so the shares were heavily over-subscribed. Many important people bought them, including Madame Dubarry. She had a private Mesmer apparatus by her bedside, but complained: "The fee demanded by this doctor for explaining the use of his magnetic apparatus was no less than one hundred *louis*, and it surprised me, nay, shook my faith, that the man who declared his sole object was to serve humanity should have expected so vast a sum from his supporters."[13]

32

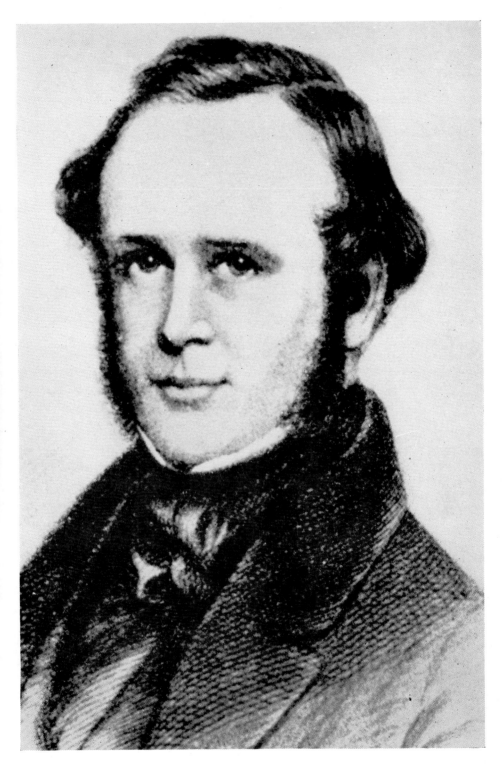

Portrait of Horace Wells

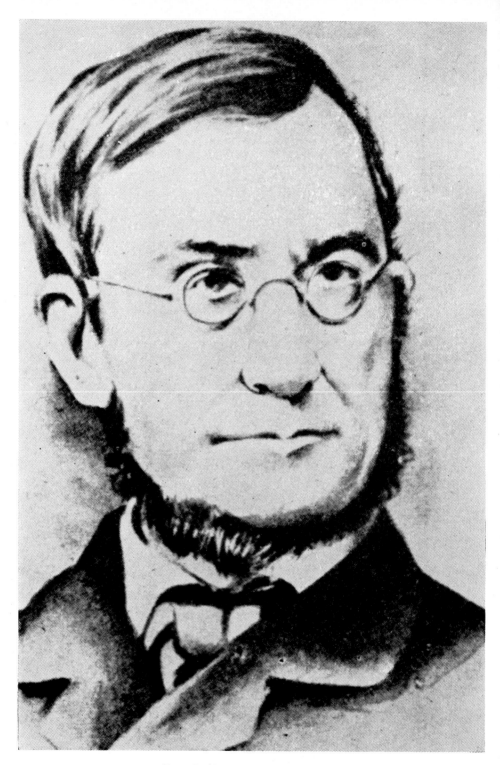

Portrait of Professor Charles Jackson

The Revolution soon cut short the controversy, and many of Mesmer's most famous patients became the victims of Dr Guillotin's new humane killer. Mesmer had to flee from France, but his name still lingered on in some parts of Europe. One of his disciples, Count Maxime de Puységur, made a startling discovery. He had a magnetized lime-tree in his park, and when his peasants were ill they came there to be cured. One day a shepherd was tied to the tree, and the Count was making the usual passes over his body when instead of the expected crisis the man fell into a profound sleep. The Count ordered him to untie himself. The man did so and started to walk away although his eyes were still firmly shut. The Count then found that whatever orders he gave, they were always promptly obeyed by the man. He went round giving demonstrations of his behaviour, and soon the news spread through Europe. In spite of official opposition a few doctors adopted the method to try to relieve their patients' pain, and Dr John Elliotson, a friend of the novelist Thackeray, declared that God in his infinite mercy had implanted in the human body the healing power of animal magnetism and that it was much more effective than any narcotics. He was so firmly convinced that this method could be used to provide painless surgery that he resigned from his post at University College Hospital to devote himself solely to the task of applying the sleep induced by this mesmerism to the field of operative surgery.

Throughout the world patients begged their doctors to use mesmerism to ease their pain, and the doctors in their turn pressed for a proper scientific investigation. An official inquiry was begun, and operations were performed under mesmerism by Strohmeyer in Vienna, by Nelaton in France, and in Boston at the Massachusetts General Hospital by John Collins Warren, the famous American surgeon who was later to play such an immense part in Morton's own story. In every case mesmerism failed to prevent even the pain of the first incision, the patients screamed as usual, and the method was completely discredited. *The Lancet* declared it to be nothing but a preposterous humbug which no one could possibly take seriously, and said that practitioners using it should be expelled from the profession as quacks and swindlers.

The intense interest aroused throughout the world, the publicity which surrounded mesmerism, and the devotion of its disciples made the final shock when it was officially proved a failure all the greater. Millions who had believed in it and clung to it like drowning men to a rope were thrust back by its failure, disillusioned and disgusted. For men like Morton it left behind a legacy of scepticism. Doctors were contemptuous and ready to condemn any means of preventing pain as humbug and the man promoting it as a charlatan. Medical authorities everywhere held that pain was an inevitable part of life and attempts to alleviate it useless. But Morton refused to accept this view; he read, he searched, he experimented. Every day in the hospital he listened to lectures, examined patients, talked to his teachers, hoping one day to glean somewhere a clue which would lead him to an efficient pain-killer. Mrs Morton says: "At the time of our marriage Dr Morton was twenty-four years old . . . and his mind was already occupied with thoughts destined to lead to his discovery. Every spare hour he could get was spent in experiment."[14]

At home with Jackson Morton discussed the problems he was constantly encountering in his delicate dental work. One day, when he was asking Jackson about teeth which had been treated with arsenic to destroy the nerves and said he was doubtful whether such teeth could be restored to usefulness because the arsenic produced an irritation and left a soreness, often permanent, Jackson recommended Morton to try his toothache drops to deaden the pain. These turned out to be pure ether, and he told Morton about students pouring ether on their handkerchiefs and inhaling it until it made them reel and stagger.

This was in July 1844, and a few days later Morton tried out the ether which Jackson had given him on a Miss Parrot from Gloucester, Massachusetts, who came to consult him. When he found the pain was more than she could bear he applied to the tooth a little sulphuric ether to deaden the pain. She called several times on subsequent days, and each time he applied the ether with the same success. One day, having kept her rather longer than usual and used it a little more freely, he was surprised to find how completely the surrounding parts had been numbed. The idea then occurred to him that if the whole system could in some way be brought under its influence, perhaps the effect could be extended and used to relieve more intense pain.

Here then was the art of the real discoverer, for from this one observation Morton suddenly saw that ether might have a universal application and made the leap from established knowledge into the realm of the unknown. All great discoverers have had this extraordinary ability to recognize what everyone else sees merely as an isolated instance as having much greater significance, and quite simple happenings point the way for them to great theories. When Galileo saw the lamps swinging in the cathedral at Pisa he started formulating his theories about the pendulum and oscillations. For Newton it was the falling fruit which set him off on a line of thought about moving bodies and gravity. Although other people must have seen these things hundreds of times before, it took a man of genius to recognize their significance.

So it was with Morton. Jackson and thousands of other doctors and scientists had often used ether, but only Morton realized its potentialities, for suddenly it dawned on him that ether might provide the answer he was seeking. But how was the ether to be applied? He could not immerse a patient's whole body in ether. Perhaps there was some way it could be washed over sufficiently and consistently to produce numbness? He was so excited about the possibilities of ether as a pain-killer that right away he started a series of experiments with it. But by now it was stifling hot in Boston, and Morton had caught 'summer fever'. To recover from this and to allow himself more time for experimenting Morton left the city and went to stay at his father-in-law's house in Farmington. He took with him some of Dr Jackson's library and other books on this subject. He asked his brother-in-law, Francis Whitman, to get him some chloric ether and immediately started a series of experiments upon birds and animals, but without much success. His friends laughed at him about his experiments, and he says: "These experiments produced no satisfactory result, and they being known among my friends, I was mortified and vexed, and bottled up the subjects where they remain to this day."[15]

Morton came back again to Boston in the autumn of 1844, fully recovered from his bout of fever, but disillusioned by the failure of his experiments with ether. His practice had fallen behind, his medical studies were lagging, and he had to work very hard to catch up. He was so busy that he had no time for further experiments, but still he believed that somewhere in the world there was a way of deadening pain, and that some day he would find it.

NOTES TO CHAPTER III

1. *McClure's Magazine*, September 1896.
2. *Ibid.*
3. *Ibid.*
4. *Ibid.*
5. *Ibid.*
6. Nathan Rice, *Trials of a Public Benefactor*.
7. *Ibid.*
8. *Ibid.*
9. *Ibid.*
10. Margaret Goldsmith, *Franz Anton Mesmer*.
11. *Ibid.*
12. *Ibid.*
13. *Ibid.*
14. *McClure's Magazine*, September 1896.
15. Nathan Rice, *op. cit.*

CHAPTER

IV

WHEN a search has been going on for hundreds of years the actual discovery always seems miraculous, as if the darkness has suddenly been pierced by a brilliant light. Yet many may have spent their lives groping towards the final truth, each generation building upon the shoulders of its fathers. For Morton much of the groundwork had already been accomplished by men like Priestley, Davy, and Hickman. Priestley discovered oxygen, and wrote about it: "Who can tell but that, in time, this pure air may become a fashionable article of luxury? Hitherto only two mice and myself have had the privilege of breathing it."[1]

Priestley also discovered several other gases, including nitrous oxide, and Davy carried on where he had left off, trying out nitrous oxide on himself, a whiff at a time. He noted a feeling of lightness in his body, a relaxation of the muscles, and an agreeableness to the point where he actually broke out laughing, and because of this property nitrous oxide also became known as 'laughing gas'. Doctors became interested, and 'pneumatic medicine' soon became popular, with gases being used in the treatment of disorders of the respiratory system and even for treating scurvy and cancer. At Dr Beddoes's pneumatic institute at Clifton Davy prepared a chemically pure nitrous oxide which was less risky, and constructed almost impermeable silk bags to hold it. He tried the gas out on his friends, and, as today, writers were among the first to volunteer. Samuel Taylor Coleridge wrote: "I experienced the most voluptuous sensations. The outer world grew dim, and I had the most entrancing visions. For three and a half minutes I lived in a world of new sensations."[2] Patients declared that they had been "born again", and some young ladies that "Mr Davy's silk bags hold the key to Paradise".[3]

The inhaling of ether vapour was also recommended. Discovered by the

36

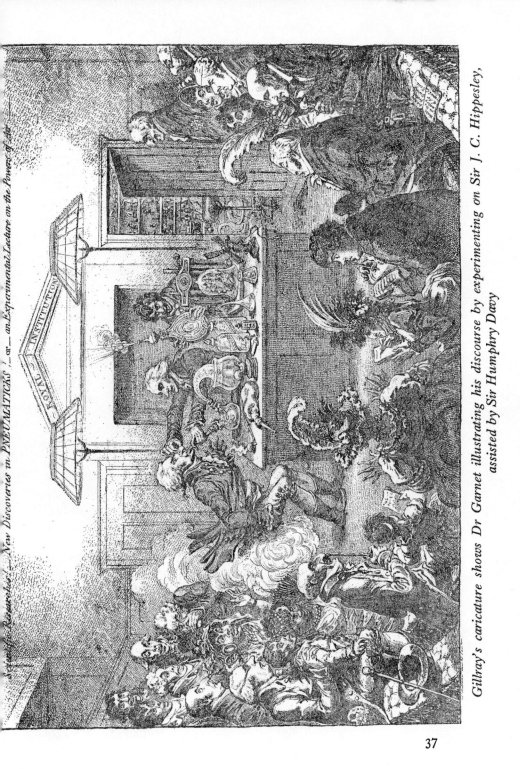

Gillray's caricature shows Dr Garnet illustrating his discourse by experimenting on Sir J. C. Hippesley, assisted by Sir Humphry Davy

37

alchemist Raymond Lully in the thirteenth century, the "sweet vitriol" he described had been completely forgotten and had then to be rediscovered again two centuries later by Paracelsus: "Of all the extracts of vitriol, this particular one is the most important, being stable. Furthermore, it has an agreeable taste, so that even chickens take it gladly, and thereafter fall asleep for a long time, awaking undamaged. In view of the effect of this vitriol, I think it especially noteworthy that its use may be recommended for painful illnesses, and that it will mitigate the disagreeable complications of these." It seems extraordinary that none of the doctors or scientists took his suggestion farther, and its potentialities remained unnoticed until Morton made his great discovery. But ether was at any rate hailed by the pneumatologists as another great cure. Maupassant used it, and says in *Sur l'Eau*: "Migraine is atrocious torment, one of the worst in the world, weakening the nerves, driving one mad, scattering one's thoughts to the winds and impairing the memory. So terrible are these headaches that I can do nothing but lie on a couch and try to dull the pain by sniffing ether."

But in spite of the pneumatologists there had always been a considerable body of opinion which regarded gases as highly dangerous, and, in fact, an American, Dr Lantham Mitchell, who tried out nitrous oxide on animals and nearly killed them, concluded that it was a powerful poison, and even that it was the semi-mythical contagium by which epidemic diseases were spread. Now doubts began to creep in. Doctors became concerned about the dangers, for they had noticed a slowing down of the pulses in their patients, and attacks of giddiness and unconsciousness were reported. It was the same story as mesmerism all over again, for the enthusiasm turned as quickly into antagonism, and advocates of pneumatic medicine were openly denounced as charlatans. At length the inhalation of laughing gas was made illegal in England, and poor Dr Beddoes was compelled to turn his institute into a hospital. In 1808, on his death-bed, he wrote to Davy: "Greetings from Dr Beddoes, one who has scattered abroad the Avena Fatua of knowledge, from which neither branch nor blossom nor fruit has resulted."[4] And when Hickman reported the reaction of animals to various gases he was ridiculed and dismissed as a madman.

Nevertheless these were the men to whom Morton owed a great debt, and after him the world. But unfortunately, although great strides had been made by the discovery and use of these gases, fear had continually crept in, fear about what exactly was their effect on patients, fear of the state of unconsciousness which resulted from their use. Each time a patient became unconscious doctors believed that they had unlocked the door to death, and, indeed, in many cases they had, for there were deaths as a result of using gases, as there are even today in hospitals and dental surgeries. Again, just when a breakthrough might have been made the doctors became scared and, again, what had been so eagerly snatched up as a cure for all pains was as quickly dropped. Gases were thrown aside by scientists in favour of other subjects, much was forgotten, and logical lines of thought were abandoned.

As ether had been forgotten and had to be rediscovered, so its effects had to be slowly and painfully brought to light again by Morton more than twenty years later, for the inhalation of gases lingered on only to provide fun for medical students and people inhaling for 'kicks'. But had it not been for these amusing effects the inhalation of gases might easily have lapsed entirely into oblivion. The medical profession has always shown an inclination towards laughter, perhaps to counteract the macabre and gruesome nature of the work, and teachers in medical schools used to amuse their students by giving them ether and nitrous oxide to inhale. Their ridiculous antics enlivened otherwise dull lectures, and the students themselves continued the fun after lessons. In America, where alcohol was almost totally forbidden, private ether parties or 'frolics' became quite popular.

What was at first fun for medical students was soon exploited by showmen. These were the great days for travelling showmen in the United States, and they quickly seized on laughing gas to provide a cheap and easy form of entertainment. In Puritan America, where card-playing, the theatre, circuses, and other entertainments of the Old World were regarded as devices of the devil, there were large audiences of settlers and immigrants uprooted from their usual haunts and friends, with time and money to spare and anxious to be amused. By advertising the fun as scientific lectures the showman avoided the puritanical censorship. He arrived usually in the new town wheeling a portable laboratory on a handcart, borrowed a table from the nearest tavern, set up his apparatus, and started his 'lecture'. First he used his megaphone to draw the crowds, and then began to perform a few simple experiments to make liquids change colour or to produce small explosions to amuse his audience. In bigger towns the more successful operators hired halls, advertised in local newspapers, printed handbills, engaged barkers, and so on. It was an advertisement for one of these lectures appearing in the *Hartford Courant* one day in December 1844 which caught the eye of Morton's former dental partner, Horace Wells:

A GRAND EXHIBITION of the effects produced by inhaling NITROUS OXIDE, EXHILARATING *or* LAUGHING GAS! will be given at Union Hall this Tuesday Evening, December 10, 1844. . . .

Forty Gallons of The Gas will be prepared and administered to all in the audience who desire to inhale it. . . .

Twelve Young Men have volunteered to inhale the gas to commence the entertainment.

Eight Strong Men are engaged to occupy the front seats, to protect

39

those under the influence of the gas from injuring themselves or others. This course is adopted that no apprehension of danger may be entertained. Probably no one will attempt to fight. . . .

N.B. The gas will be administered only to gentlemen of the first respectability. The object is to make the *entertainment in every respect, a genteel affair.* . . .

The entertainment is *scientific* to those who make it *scientific.* . . .

No language can describe the delightful sensation produced. Robert Southey (poet) once said that the atmosphere of the highest of all heavens must be composed of the Gas. . . .

For a full account of the effect produced upon some of the most distinguished men of Europe, see Hooper's Medical Dictionary. . . . The History and properties of the Gas will be explained at the commencement of the entertainment. . . .

The entertainment will close with a few of the most surprising chemical experiments.

Mr Colton will give a private entertainment to those Ladies who desire to inhale the Gas, Tuesday between 12 and 1 o'clock, free. None but Ladies will be admitted. . . .

Entertainment to commence at 7 o'clock.

Tickets 25 cents.[5]

The exhibition was given by Gardner Quincy Colton, and Wells went along with his wife, Liza, and all the other "best people" to the Union Hall to enjoy this "genteel affair". Colton opened with an amusing account of the gas, and then, to encourage the audience, he appeared to inhale a considerable quantity of it himself from a rubber bag. He was a clever showman and started to declaim, his words rolling out in a glorious stream. Suddenly he stopped, put his hand to his head, and announced solemnly, "The effect is now nearly gone." He then invited volunteers to come up on the stage to perform.

At a further private demonstration arranged for the following morning one of the volunteers was Samuel Cooley, a young man who worked in a drug-store in Hartford. Hardly had he started to inhale before he began to dance about like a lunatic. Sitting near was an assistant in a rival drug-store, and at Cooley's antics he burst out laughing. When Cooley caught sight of him his high spirits turned to fury. Plunging into the hall, he chased after his derider from bench to bench, and row to row, right through the hall. Under the effects of the gas he continually crashed into the benches, knocking them down, and himself too. Each time, apparently unaware of any pain, he was soon on his feet again. Then, as the effects of the gas began to pass off, he came to a stop and stood there looking round in bewilderment and smiling ruefully, not far from Horace Wells. The gentlemen present were highly amused and excited at his antics, but Wells was puzzled. He knew Cooley had struck himself severely several times, but he did not seem to feel any pain. Wells went over to ask if he had not

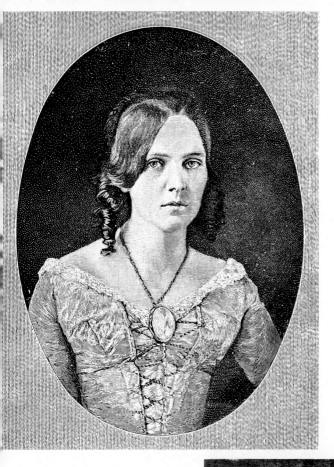

Portrait of
Mrs William Morton,
aged eighteen

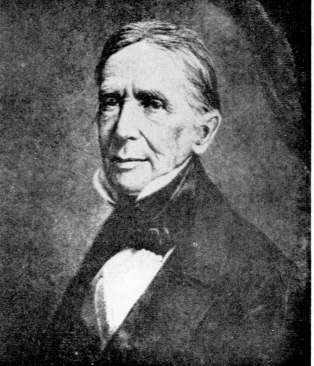

Professor
John C. Warren

A GRAND EXHIBITION

OF THE EFFECTS PRODUCED BY INHALING

NITROUS OXIDE, EXHILERATING, OR

LAUGHING GAS!

WILL BE GIVEN AT *the Masonic Hall*

Saturday EVENING, *15*th   1845.

10 GALLONS OF GAS will be prepared and administered to all in the audience who desire to inhale it.

MEN will be invited from the audience, to protect those under the influence of the Gas from injuring themselves or others. This course is adopted that no apprehension of danger may be entertained. Probably no one will attempt to fight.

THE EFFECT OF THE GAS is to make those who inhale it, either

LAUGH, SING, DANCE, SPEAK OR FIGHT, &c. &c.

according to the leading trait of their character. They seem to retain consciousness enough not to say or do that which they would have occasion to regret.

N. B. The Gas will be administered only to gentlemen of the first respectability. The object is to make the entertainment in every respect, a genteel affair.

Those who inhale the Gas once, are always anxious to inhale it the second time. There is not an exception to this rule.

No language can describe the delightful sensation produced. Robert Southey, (poet) once said that "the atmosphere of the highest of all possible heavens must be composed of this Gas."

For a full account of the effect produced upon some of the most distinguished men of Europe, see Hooper's Medical Dictionary, under the head of Nitrogen.

The History and properties of the Gas will be explained at the commencement of the entertainment.

The entertainment will be accompanied by experiments in

ELECTRICITY.

ENTERTAINMENT TO COMMENCE AT 7 O'CLOCK.

TICKETS *12½* CENTS,

Poster advertising an exhibition of laughing gas

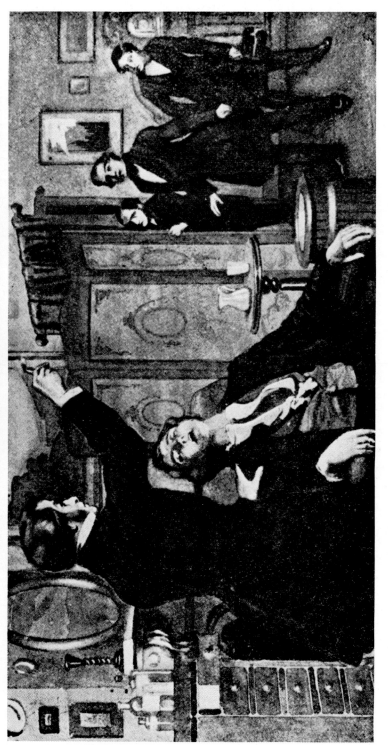

"A new era in tooth-pulling." Wells has one of his own teeth extracted under the influence of nitrous oxide

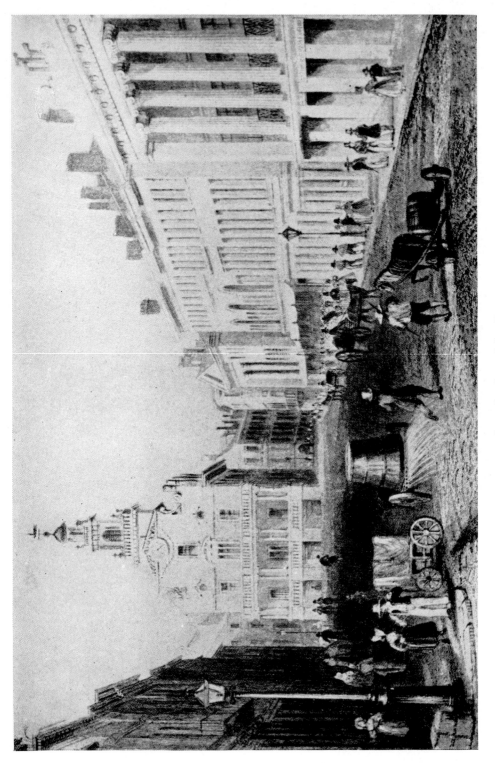

Boston, about the time of the discovery

hurt himself. Only then did Cooley pull up his trouser-legs to see. There he saw to his amazement several severe bruises, cuts, and abrasions. Wells explained that he had fallen over some of the benches. Still Cooley could hardly believe it.

There are several versions of what happened in these demonstrations, and in later years Wells used to tell how he fidgeted on the edge of his chair, waiting impatiently for the effects of the gas to wear off so that he could ply Cooley with questions about his injury. Did he really not know he had done it? Had he no recollection? Was there no sense of pain from it? Wells was certainly extraordinarily excited, and told Colton that after seeing Cooley cut his leg without any sensation of pain he "believed that a person could have a tooth extracted while under its influence and not feel any pain".[6] Colton warned him that the effects of the gas were by no means certain. Still Wells argued that it was bound to work and that he was sure he was going to be able to make a fortune from it. He even offered Colton a share of the business if he would come in with him and be responsible for administering the gas. Still Colton hesitated; the nitrous oxide would not be sufficiently powerful, it was not entirely safe, and he was not keen to have anything to do with Wells's mad scheme. Wells retorted that he was sure it would be successful, and what was more, that he would prove it: he would have one of his own teeth taken out with the gas, and that would settle it!

Wells got hold of a colleague of his, John Mankey Riggs, who had assisted Wells from time to time in his practice and was himself to become well known as the discoverer of alveolar pyorrhoea, named after him 'Riggs' disease'. Riggs was very sceptical about the powers of nitrous oxide, but Wells finally persuaded him to do the extraction, and Wells, Riggs, Colton, and his brother all assembled in Wells's surgery. Wells sat down in the dental chair, and Colton put the mouthpiece of the gasbag between his lips, holding the wooden tap ready to release the gas. Wells looked utterly confident, but the others were nervous and afraid. Prudently Riggs went to the door and set it open, so that they would be able to escape quickly in case Wells became ill or raving mad or died in the chair. Riggs said afterwards their agreement was to push the administration to a point never reached before. They did not know whether death or success confronted them. It was a *terra incognita* they were bound to explore.

Wells took a deep breath of the gas, coughed briefly, then continued inhaling with slow, regular breaths. His face, usually pale, went ashen, and his lips turned blue. Immediately Riggs picked up the dental forceps, reached in for the tooth, and extracted it. Wells's eyes were glazed over, and as Riggs released his head it fell forward on to his chest. Riggs bent down to him to see whether his heart was still beating. Was he dead? Still Wells did not stir. Riggs looked round at the circle. No one said a word.

41

They were all staring intently at Wells's face, terror-stricken. Suddenly they all made a rush towards the door, but, just at that moment, Wells began to move. His hands fluttered a moment, and he began to breathe more naturally. He opened his eyes, and was so startled when he saw the tooth he exclaimed triumphantly, "A new era in tooth-pulling!" As they all crowded round he told them how he had not felt "as much as the prick of a pin".

Wells was soon dancing about the room, talking wildly about opening up a practice for painless extractions immediately and how they would all make their fortunes from it. Colton and Riggs begged him not to rush into things, and reminded him of the dangers. In fact, they were almost as excited as Wells, but tried to persuade him to be cautious. Eventually Riggs was able to convince Wells that patients would need some assurance about the gas, its safety as well as its efficacy, and insisted Wells must get some scientist, someone of standing who would support his claim, someone like Professor Charles Jackson. Wells had already applied to him two years before for a certificate of approval for his dental solder, and they agreed that if Jackson could be persuaded to give his name in support of the new treatment they would be home and dry.

Wells knew his previous partner, William Morton, was boarding with Jackson, and decided to approach Jackson through him. Morton consented, and they saw him together on January 17th, 1845. Wells triumphantly described to Jackson how he had used nitrous oxide and had extracted the tooth without pain, and Jackson listened condescendingly to what he had to say. At the end Wells waited eagerly for some word of approval, but instead Jackson turned on him scornfully and ordered him imperiously to go no farther with his crazy experiments. Throughout the ages, he told them, man had dreamed of overcoming pain. Everything had been tried—herbs, drugs, faith, mesmerism, alcohol—but all in vain. It was no good looking for a pain-killer, for there was no such thing, and, like Copland, he took the view that "even were the reports of persons who felt no pain during an operation credible, this would not be worth the consideration of a serious-minded doctor". Scientists knew that pain was an inevitable part of life, and it was not for mere dentists to attempt to question established scientific theories. To do so would almost certainly discredit Wells, and even lay him open to a charge of manslaughter. He ordered Wells to give up such nonsense immediately, and with that he brusquely dismissed the pair of them.

Wells stalked out, furious at what he considered to be Jackson's offhand treatment. He was still convinced that he would have great success with laughing gas, and was determined somehow to get it officially tested. He would go, he said, to the Massachusetts General Hospital, to John Collins Warren no less. Warren would surely recognize the greatness of his discovery. But not for a moment did he consider his position, or the facts of his case, for he had tried out nitrous oxide on no more than a handful of patients, and even so had succeeded in only about half of them. Impulsive and impatient as usual, Wells went straight off to Warren to ask for a chance to demonstrate his painless extraction. Warren was used to such foolish claims, backed by little scientific proof and a lot of enthusiasm, but agreed to the gas being demonstrated before a class of his medical students. "His students", said Morton, "were preparing to inhale that very evening for sport, and he offered to announce the purpose to them and ask them to meet us at the college. In the evening Dr Wells and myself went to the hall and I took my instruments."[7]

When the time came Warren's voice was full of sarcasm as he introduced Wells to the students: "There is a gentleman here who purports to have something which will destroy pain in surgical operations. He wants to address you. If any of you would like to hear him, you are at liberty to do so."[8]

Wells stepped forward, his chubby face gleaming with excitement. One of the Harvard students who had an aching tooth and had volunteered to be a guinea-pig sat waiting in the chair. Wells was very flustered and kept fumbling and dropping the instruments, but at last managed to give him the gas. Taking up his forceps, he got a firm grip on the tooth, but as he started to pull, the victim let out a terrified yell, and all the students began to laugh and hiss. "Humbug!" they shouted. "A swindle!" For a moment the whole room was in an uproar, and poor Wells fled, leaving his instruments behind him. According to Morton, "the spectators laughed and hissed when the patient screamed from pain. The meeting broke up and we were looked upon as having made ourselves very ridiculous."[9]

Wells left Boston the following morning to return home to Hartford. Here he arranged a further demonstration, but this time he gave too large a dose and the patient almost died. Then and there he decided to give up, and on February 5th, 1845, his house was advertised as to let in the *Hartford Courant*. Afterwards he announced that he had temporarily given up his practice due to ill-health, and recommended to his patients his friend and assistant, John Riggs. Disheartened and disappointed by his failure, he dropped it all as quickly as he had picked it up, for Wells was an ebullient character, always eager to take up new ideas, but without the necessary patience and application to see them through. He had rushed headlong into the demonstration, without sufficient experience, without sufficient preparation, and although he had been quick to recognize the potentialities of laughing gas, he did not stick at it long enough to work out the vast problems involved.

With hard work and serious experiment Wells might have realized that the amount he gave at the hospital was only enough to elate the patient,

43

not to produce that solid state of unconsciousness needed to extract teeth painlessly. But he would also have had to establish that if anything but the purest gas is given the patient behaves crazily, that the patient becomes cyanosed first, and that each patient presents a different problem. Above all, he would have had to discover that the use of oxygen diminishes the unpredictability, and he would have to have gone on and devised a much better apparatus. In fact, it took a quarter of a century before dentists were able to perfect a method of using nitrous oxide, even for the painless extraction of teeth.

So Wells chose to throw it all up. He left dentistry altogether and set to arranging a panorama of natural history for the city hall in Hartford. After this he became a bird fancier and travelled through Connecticut with a troupe of singing canaries, visiting one town after another, giving shows and trying to sell birds. But this did not provide money quickly enough for him, and he moved on to something new again. This time it was selling shower-baths. Americans were becoming sophisticated urban dwellers, and Wells thought that there was a great market for shower-baths. He travelled round trying to sell patented baths and coal-sifters, but this did not provide much of a living either. Engravings and paintings were next, and he went hurrying off to Europe. Here then was the very chance he had been looking for: he would buy them there cheaply and bring them back to America and sell them for a fortune . . . and so it went on. Life for Wells continued always in this erratic fashion; seizing on each thing with enormous enthusiasm, he was always ready to exploit a new line of business, always ready to take up catchpenny schemes, but certainly with none of the makings of a scientist who must depend more on solid proof than haphazard discovery. He had great imagination, but not the ability for hard work which goes to make a genius.

But what Wells lacked Morton had in abundance. His capacity for hard and painstaking work was phenomenal. He had already carried out experiments himself with ether, and although Wells's disastrous demonstration disappointed him, it had made him even more aware of the tremendous problem which had to be solved. And it was to these problems that he now devoted himself.

NOTES TO CHAPTER IV

1. Joseph Priestley, *Experiments and Observations on Different Kinds of Air* (London, 1775).
2. T. E. Thorpe, *Humphry Davy* (London, 1896).
3. *Ibid.*
4. John E. Stock, *Memoirs of the Life of Thomas Beddoes*, M.D., 1811.

5. *Hartford Courant*, December 10th, 1844.
6. United States, 32nd Congress, 2nd Session in the Senate of the United States, February 19th, 1853.
7. Nathan Rice, *Trials of a Public Benefactor*.
8. *Ibid*.
9. *Ibid*.

CHAPTER

V

IT is an extraordinary thing that, although men may have been searching for a discovery for thousands of years, often several people come within reach of the solution at the same time. But sometimes the work has not been brought to fruition, its merits have never been fully realized, and as far as humanity is concerned the discovery might as well never have been made. When Jenner became famous for his vaccination in 1796 a yeoman farmer named Jesty who lived in the next county announced that many years before Jenner he had taken a stocking needle and scratched cowpox material into the skins of his wife and children and had later proved their immunity by following it with material taken from a smallpox case. He had then taken no more interest in the subject until he heard that Jenner was to be given £10,000. With the help of his Member of Parliament and the village clergyman Jesty sent letters to the Jennerian Society in London to try to substantiate his claim to the discovery. He was invited to London, but, while Jenner eventually got £37,000, was presented to the kings of Europe, and had every possible honour showered upon him, all Jesty got was a portrait of himself and a pair of gold-mounted needles presented to him as a souvenir of his exploit. Although Jesty had carried out his experiment twenty years before Jenner, quite rightly he is given no credit because he had not bothered to take the matter farther than his own family. For it is only a man of genius like Jenner or Morton who appreciates the real importance of what he has discovered and perseveres until it becomes part of accepted practice.

In the case of ether, while Morton was working hard in the North, away in the Southern States of America a doctor named Long got very near to making a breakthrough, but with no idea of the importance of what he had stumbled upon. Crawford Williamson Long practised in Jefferson, a village deep in Georgia, a hundred and forty miles from the

46

nearest railway and surrounded by huge cotton plantations. It began—as with Wells—with a demonstration of laughing gas in the winter of 1841. Long had been called out to attend a patient and had been unable to see the show. His friends had missed him and went to his house to wait for him to come home. When he returned they welcomed him uproariously, hardly giving him time to get out of the saddle before telling him all that had happened. They besieged him with questions and asked why he could not give them as much fun: "You're supposed to be a doctor and know something about chemistry," they said. "Make us some gas and we'll go on a fine tear."[1]

Long went off into his surgery and brought back a bottle of ether, saturated a handkerchief, and thrust it beneath their noses. At once they began to talk nonsense, to laugh, and to dance and sing. Long, who had grown familiar with ether during his days as a student, looked on with amusement. As he bade them good-night he told them, "You see, your doctor here in Jefferson can give as good measure as any stranger."[2]

Next day they called on him and begged him to repeat the experiment, and after that on two or three evenings each week they would gather at the young doctor's house and have ether 'frolics'. The young ladies too were anxious not to be left out of the fun and begged the doctor to let them try. The tall, handsome doctor was a favourite with the girls and agreed to give them an ether party as well. He sent off a letter to Robert Goodman, a friend who kept a drug-store in Athens, Georgia, to ask for fresh supplies:

DEAR BOB,
    I am under the necessity of troubling you a little. I am entirely out of ether and wish some by tomorrow night if it is possible to receive it by that time. We have some girls in Jefferson who are anxious to see it taken, and you know nothing would afford me more pleasure than to take it in their presence and to get a few sweet kisses (?) . . . if you can meet with the opportunity to send the medicines to me tomorrow you will confer a great favour by doing so. If you cannot send them to-morrow, get Dr Reese to send them by the stage on Wednesday, I can persuade the girls to remain until Wednesday night, but would prefer receiving the ether sooner.
                                                    Your friend,
                                                    CRAWFORD LONG[3]

When the time came Long told the girls that he had brought the drug, but had decided not to inhale after all, for there was no telling what he might do while under its influence. But of course, as he had intended, the girls insisted. "All right," said Long, "I'll inhale some if you all promise not to hold me responsible for anything I may do."[4] The doctor boarded with two elderly sisters. They were both strict Quakers who would not have understood the joke at all, so he was careful first to lock the door to

47

his room. Then, with the utmost solemnity, Long poured the liquid on to a towel, put it to his face, and pretending to be a sleepwalker he marched gravely round the room kissing every girl in turn. Telling of this prank as an old man, he would slap his thigh and roar with laughter: "The girls must have liked it for they were so anxious to try the drug themselves."[5] It was one of these beautiful young girls he eventually married, and later she described him: "I yet see him, dressed in a light blue summer suit, collars and cuffs black, tan-coloured silk gloves, wide-brimmed white hat, sitting superbly on his dapple-grey charger, firm, dignified—he rides like one to command."[6]

But as well as being a dandy Long was also quite a clever man. He had graduated brilliantly at the age of nineteen and had studied medicine at both the leading schools—Transylvania and the University of Pennsylvania. After several of the ether parties he was surprised to find he had bruised himself, but had no recollection of having done so, and when one of the young men who was very fond of inhaling was afraid to have two small tumours removed because of the pain Long suggested he should take ether instead of the usual alcohol. The operation took about five minutes, and the patient, James Venables, appeared to feel nothing while the tumours were being removed from the back of his neck. Long later proved that it was no fluke by amputating two badly damaged fingers of a Negro boy, removing one with ether and one without. The boy screamed desperately and had to be strapped down for one operation, but appeared to be sleeping quietly during the other.

Long might have continued, but after using ether for only eight operations the doctors of the neighbourhood complained of his reckless behaviour, saying that they knew from their years of experience that he was bound to kill someone sooner or later. Rumours began to fly round the district that Long was using an extremely dangerous poison which put people to sleep so that he could carve them to pieces without their knowing. Soon his patients began to avoid him. Children believed he was bewitched and scuttled indoors when he came by. Old crones crossed themselves or reached for the Bible for protection against his evil eye. His practice dwindled, and even his friends began to avoid him. Eventually the village elders called on him to insist that he give up these devilish practices, and threatened that if he did not stop he would be lynched.

So, with success within his grasp, Long gave up. Like Wells, he might have gone on with his experiments and eventually given the world one of its greatest discoveries. But he too failed. Without even writing to the medical journals to make his experiments public—not realizing the importance of his discovery—the antagonism and the pressure of public opinion proved too much for him. He had no idea what he had stumbled across and soon forgot all about his few experiments. So it was left to William Morton to make the final breakthrough. All the others had tried

48

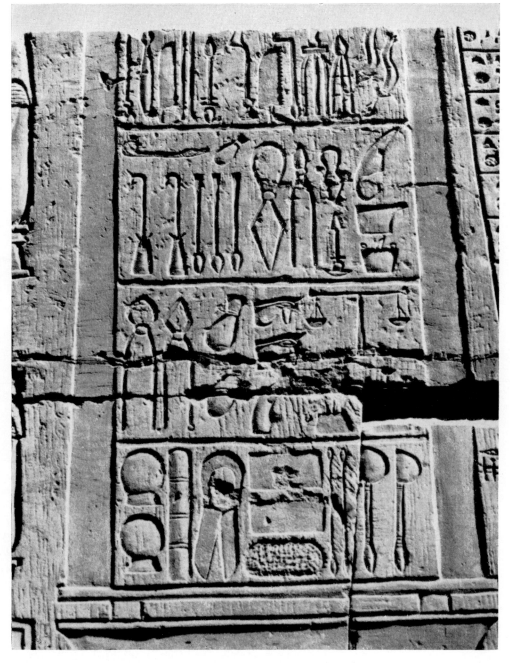

The earliest record of medical instruments, at Kom Ombo, Egypt

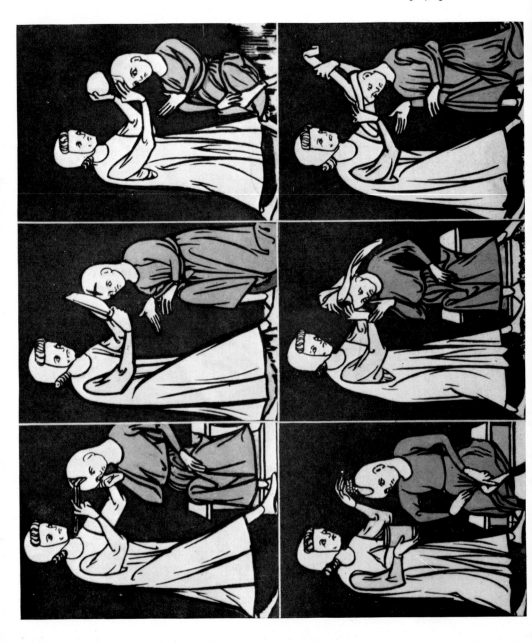

Trepanning, from a thirteenth-century treatise on surgery

and failed. Only he had the genius, the capacity for hard work, the tenacity, and the courage.

Up to now Morton had been boarding with Dr Jackson, discussing scientific problems with him at every opportunity, and making full use of his laboratory and library. He had tried hard to get on well with him, but unfortunately Jackson was a very strange man. He was thirty-nine, a tall, muscular, square-jawed man with sharp features and an extraordinary rim of straggling dark whiskers fringing his clean-shaven face like a collar. He had a forbidding appearance and was distinctly odd-looking, with "steel-rimmed spectacles placed cock-eyed on his nose, as though he did not have the time or patience to adjust them properly. . . . His face had a hard, frozen quality, as if the jaws, the muscles under the skin were held too tense, masking some explosive force inside. And yet, this look breaking up, he could be suddenly affable, his eyes glowing, his voice warm."

Jackson had studied medicine at Harvard, but had become more interested in chemistry, mineralogy, and geology. He studied at the Sorbonne in Paris and became friendly with Élie de Beaumont, the celebrated French geologist who first put forward the theory of the formation of mountains. When Jackson got back to America in 1833 he had set up practice in Boston as a doctor, but with such an unpleasant personality few patients ever stayed with him long. That year an army doctor, William Beaumont, published an account of an extraordinary medical case. Some ten years before he had been called in to attend a young man named St Martin who had the most terrible gunshot wounds. Beaumont did what he could to clean them up and then waited for the patient to die. But instead he survived miraculously, and after four months his tissues began to expel the shot, wadding, and bone splinters still left in his body. The inflammation eventually cleared up, but he was left with a hole in his stomach permanently open to the air. Beaumont immediately realized that this presented him with a unique opportunity to study the workings of the man's stomach, something which had never been done before. He wrote: "I can look directly into the cavity of the stomach, observe its motion, and almost see the process of digestion. I can pour in water with a funnel and put in food with a spoon, and draw them out again with a siphon. . . ."[7] He did more than that; he attached pieces of food to a thread and then lowered them into the poor man's stomach, withdrawing them every few minutes to see how the digestion was getting on. At one time he used "a plug of raw beef, instead of lint, to stop the orifice, and found that in less than five hours it had been completely digested off, as smooth and even as if it had been cut with a knife."[8]

It was a horrifying series of experiments which certainly advanced medical knowledge enormously, but for poor St Martin it was a terrifying life. He was expected to work as Beaumont's servant to pay for his keep, and eventually he could stand it no longer and ran away. But having very little strength he was unable to do his old job of fur-trapping properly, and after a few years, in abject poverty and nearly starving, he was forced to crawl back and subject himself once again to a further series of tests.

Beaumont made altogether some two hundred experiments on him and drew fifty "inferences", as he called them. He toured the United States and exhibited him like a circus sideshow as the "man with the window in his stomach", and Jackson saw him at the Connecticut Medical College in Boston in 1834. No one before Beaumont had ever managed to secure a pure sample of gastric juice or had any idea even what it was composed of, and Jackson begged Beaumont to let him have a phial of the fluid for analysis. But not content with that Jackson then tried to get St Martin under his control and sent a petition to the Secretary of War: "Being informed that Dr Charles T. Jackson, an eminent chemist of Boston, successfully prosecuting an analysis of the gastric fluid of Alexis St Martin, the Canadian boy attached to Dr Beaumont, surgeon of the U.S. Army . . . and regarding the case as furnishing a rare and fortunate opportunity of demonstrating important principles in physiology, by which credit may be conferred on the medical science of our country and important benefits accrue to humanity . . . and persuaded that the opportunity now afforded, if neglected, will be lost to our country for ever, we request that the Honourable Secretary of War will station Dr Beaumont at Boston. . . ."[9]

Jackson's egotism is clear as he describes himself as "an eminent chemist". He does not praise Beaumont's great series of experiments, but only calls attention to his own. The petition was signed by two hundred members of Congress and shows the measure of support that Jackson was already able to command. But in spite of his machinations he failed to take the credit from Beaumont, who had been experimenting for many years and had already published a book on this astounding case. Beaumont's discoveries in fact remained unrivalled until Pavlov began his work on digestion towards the end of the century.

But although Jackson was unsuccessful in his bid to gain control of St Martin, he soon became embroiled in a more serious claim. When Jackson came back to America in October 1832 he had sailed on the packet steamer *Sully*. On board was Samuel Morse, a portrait painter who later became famous for his electromagnetic telegraph and the Morse code named after him. Morse was a great inventor of gadgets and became dubbed the American 'Leonardo', and during the voyage he and Jackson had long talks about new magnetic devices. Morse enjoyed discussing his ideas for sending messages by electrical impulses with a keen fellow-scientist, and Jackson could be most charming when he chose. He was also good at telling stories to while away the time on what was then a long and weary journey of some weeks. But what Morse did not realize was that behind this mask of affability, beneath the façade of the helpful, dedicated scientist, lay a tortured, twisted mind. Jackson was a fiendishly jealous man whose inflated ideas of his own importance and whose deadly ambitions forced him to stop at nothing to try to steal ideas from other scientists.

When Morse returned to America he perfected his invention and set about trying to sell it. He wrote to Jackson in 1837, saying: "I called to have a long talk and tell you of the success of my telegraph."[10] Jackson sent him a puzzling reply which spoke of "our telegraph" and went on: "I have seen several notices of it, but observe my name is not connected with the discovery."[11] Morse retorted angrily: ". . . all the machinery has been elaborated without a hint from you of any kind in the remotest degree. I am the sole inventor."[12] Congress had already taken up Morse's invention, and other countries had bought licences to use it. Now when it was going to be a big success and to make Morse a wealthy man Jackson stepped in to try to claim the invention as his. A bitter controversy raged for several years, with Jackson steadfastly maintaining that he was the real inventor, insisting that on the boat Morse had no inkling of the telegraph, and that when Jackson spoke to him about electromagnetism Morse had replied, "Electromagnetism? What is it?" With exactly similar words Jackson was later to use the same manœuvre to rob another inventor of his honour.

In Morse's case Jackson was very nearly successful, for he used every possible means, petitioning Congress, the Patent Office, and the world at large to try to convince everyone that he was the true inventor of Morse's electromagnetic telegraph. He also used another tactic which was to become equally familiar, putting it about that Morse was only a mere portrait painter—an ignoramus—with no knowledge at all of science and incapable of inventing anything. In fact, this was absolutely untrue, for Morse had actually studied science at Yale, and had attended a lecture course on electromagnetism in New York University.

Morse protested at these monstrous falsehoods and spoke of Jackson as "a lunatic" and an "intolerable nuisance", but Jackson still persisted. On April 15th, 1837, Morse's brother published an article in the *New York Observer* describing an electromagnetic telegraph. Jackson immediately alleged that this was the apparatus he had detailed to Morse when they met on the *Sully*. But here he made a fatal mistake, for Samuel Morse immediately stepped in and demonstrated that this was not his telegraph, and thus proved that Jackson could have known nothing of his invention. Any normal man would have given up at this point. But Jackson was not normal. He still kept on with his campaign to claim the credit, and to everyone's astonishment in January 1839 a paragraph appeared in the *Boston Post*: "We are informed that the invention of the electromagnetic telegraph, which has been claimed by Mr S. F. B. Morse of New York, is entirely due to our fellow-citizen, Dr Charles T. Jackson, who first conceived the idea of such an instrument during his return from Europe in the packet ship *Sully* in October 1832." Jackson insisted that he had exhibited the telegraph to "a class of twenty-five ladies and one gentleman, and also to several scientific gentlemen", but when asked to name just one of them he made the excuse, "It would not be proper for me to give their names." When Morse visited Europe to try to get the British and French Governments to buy his invention Jackson wrote to all his influential friends in the French Academy of Sciences. "I regret," he said, "to see in public papers that Professor Samuel F. B. Morse has appropriated to himself my electromagnetic telegraph. . . ." Eventually Morse was able to prove Jackson a liar, but for all these seven years Jackson pursued Morse, circulating rumours about his lack of ability and scientific knowledge and claiming that the invention rightly belonged to him. He must have made Morse's life absolutely wretched, and certainly cost him a great deal of time and money defending his name and proving to Congress that he was in fact the real inventor.

While all this had been going on the subject was an obsession with Jackson. He continually talked about Morse and constantly repeated all the petty details. Morse's inexperience seemed to rile him most, for he could not bear to think that someone with less scientific education than himself should have won so much from the invention, and he harped on this all the time. It certainly must have been galling to realize that if he had only appreciated the significance of their discussions on board the *Sully* he could indeed have perfected and patented the invention himself. Jackson's megalomania made life in his household very difficult. He had a vile and uncontrollable temper at the best of times, and now it became much worse. Morton and his wife tried hard to steer the conversation away from such subjects as Morse's invention and to avoid the arguments which repeatedly blew up. But they were not always successful, and it was a most difficult and embarrassing time for both of them. At last it all came to a head. Morton acted as a lay preacher in the Congregational church and took a service there every Sunday. Week after week there was trouble when Jackson accused Morton of keeping him waiting for his dinner. Eventually one Sunday when Jackson flew into a particularly furious rage about it Morton could stand his jibes no longer, for he felt he could not expose his young wife, now expecting their first child, to any more such scenes, and they packed their bags and left.

Afterwards Morton felt sorry about the incident. He was a devout Christian and sent Jackson a letter of apology and a farewell present. On May 13th, 1845, Jackson wrote in reply:

> Accept my warm thanks for the elegant travelling case you have had the kindness to present to me. It is really too handsome for use in our backwood camps [on his geological expeditions]; but since it is your wish that it should accompany me in my wanderings, I shall take it in memory of its donor.
>
> Your obliged friend.[13]

The Mortons moved into rooms. They were rather cramped, but he managed to continue with his practice, his medical studies, and, when he had the time, with his search for a pain-killer.

One day a year later, in June 1846, he came upon the following observation in Pereira's *Elements of the Materia Medica* (London, 1839): "The vapour of ether is inhaled in spasmodic asthma, chronic catarrh, whooping cough, and dyspepsia, and to relieve the effects caused by the accidental inhalation of chlorine gas." Morton had heard of inhalation of ether for amusement, but had no idea that the inhaling could be prolonged. He was very excited and that same day said to a friend of his, Dr Augustus Gould, "I will have some way yet by which I will perform my operations without pain", to which Gould replied, "If you could effect that you would do more than human wisdom has yet done or than I expect it will ever do."[14]

But how exactly was the ether to be inhaled? Could the vapour be used like nitrous oxide? Was it entirely safe? What was the proper dose? What were the effects? Morton immediately went round asking everyone he knew for information on the subject, and a student named Spear who had just started working for him as one of his assistants described the ether parties held by the students at Lexington and how they inhaled ether to 'go high'. Morton was resolved to continue with his experiments, and talked also about his plans to Joseph Wightman, a surgical-instrument maker who afterwards became Mayor of Boston. Wightman was very impressed by Morton's resolution and told his wife, "You will see, Mary, this young dentist will be able to pull out our teeth without hurting us."[15]

But again Morton was reminded of the dangers. A pharmacist told him of a man who had lain apparently insensible for nearly two days after inhaling, and Faraday said, "By the imprudent inspiration of ether a gentleman was thrown into a lethargic state." Morton went off also to talk to Metcalf, who ran Joseph Burnett's drug-store only a few doors away at 33 Tremont Street. Metcalf was a leading druggist in the town, and he warned Morton severely of the dangers of ether, telling him it might be taken in small quantities, but "if taken in larger quantities, its effects would be dangerous and lasting, if not fatal."[16]

Morton was very worried by Metcalf's warning and sat up all night staring at the bottle of ether, wondering whether to go on or not. He bitterly regretted his lack of education, but on this there was little to guide him anyway, for it was entirely new territory. All the authorities agreed that too large a dose inevitably resulted in death, but no one knew what was a safe dose or how much caused death, or, even more important, what were the symptoms and signals before this point was reached. But everyone insisted that the patient could suddenly pass from apparent intoxication to death. After a sleepless night he made a momentous decision: he would give up his practice and devote himself entirely to experimenting. He felt sure there must be a pain-killer somewhere and that ether must eventually supply the answer, and he was now determined to find it, whatever the cost to his practice, his medical studies, and his career.

The following morning, the last day of June 1846, he went to see Grenville Hayden, a Boston dentist who was a friend of his, to ask him to superintend his practice, giving as a reason that he had an idea in his head, which he thought would be one of the greatest things ever known, and that it was something he had discovered which would enable him to extract teeth without pain. He then bought a large supply of ether from Burnett's and set off immediately with his family to his house in West Needham to embark upon a further series of experiments.

NOTES TO CHAPTER V

1. Frances Long Taylor, *Crawford W. Long and the Discovery of Ether Anaesthesia*.
2. *Ibid.*
3. J. Jacobs, *Dr Crawford W. Long*.
4. *Ibid.*
5. *Ibid.*
6. Frances Long Taylor, *op. cit.*
7. William Beaumont, *Experiments and Observations*.
8. *Ibid.*
9. Petition to Congress.
10. Amos Kendall, *Morse's patent, full exposure of Dr. Charles T. Jackson's pretensions*.
11. *Ibid.*
12. *Ibid.*
13. Nathan Rice, *Trials of a Public Benefactor*.
14. *Ibid.*
15. *Ibid.*
16. *Ibid.*

CHAPTER

VI

WHEN his practice had first begun to flourish Morton had bought forty acres of land at West Needham, what is now Wellesley, just south-west of Boston. Here, where the town hall now stands, Morton built a house—their first home—made a farm on the land that lay around it, and built a cottage for his parents. Until then they had had no proper home, for the family had been scattered when Morton's father lost all his money, and now at long last Morton was able to bring them together again. "My great object," he says, "was to make a home for my parents and sisters and I have had that satisfaction."

Mrs Hale gives her usual fulsome description of it all:

In 1845 he purchased a barren pasture, now on it is Etherton Cottage, showing once again energy and unwearied industry. . . . This cottage home . . . is about thirty miles ride from Boston on the Great Western Railroad leading from Boston to Worcester.

The grounds embrace about six acres in a natural basin surrounded by an amphitheatre of forest-clad hills dotted with residences. From the centre of this hollow rises a knoll, and on it stands the cottage (a model architecture in its style and finish)—a picturesque building of the English style of rural architecture.

The prospect from its every window is, of course, superb. In the foreground are the serpentine walks, rustic summerhouses, flowerbeds, young trees, sparkling streams and other appurtenances of the mansion itself.

Beyond we see the village church, the farm houses of the industrious yeomanry and the other quiet beauties of a country landscape, while an occasional train sweeps along the adjacent railway like a fiery dragon, a type of the nervous, go-ahead spirit of this utilitarian age.[1]

Morton was himself very much a man of this go-ahead age. His wife

55

says: "Dr Morton was one of those tremendously earnest men who believe they have a high destiny to fulfil. How many times he said to me in the months preceding his great discovery: 'I have work to do in this world, Lizzie!' Or again: 'The time will come when I will do away with pain!'"[2]

Morton's first experiments were with birds and insects, and even gold-fish. Fifty years later Mrs Morton wrote about them, how at West Needham:

> Where was our summer home, there was a spring which contained a number of goldfish, and I noticed that my husband would often go to it, and I would see him catching the fish and looking at them intently as if studying them as he held them wriggling in his hand. . . . "Do you put the fish asleep, too?" I asked, laughing. "I try to," he said, quite seriously, "but I have not succeeded yet." I laughed again, thinking it was all a joke, but my husband became very grave, and said, "The time will come, my dear, when I will banish pain from the world." It was at this time he used to bottle up all sorts of queer bugs and insects until the house was full of crawling things. He would administer ether to all these little creatures, and especially the big green worms he found on grape vines. I remember how Dr Morton's friends laughed at the queer experiments, and I am afraid I joined with them sometimes. But he continued on his way undaunted, frequently saying: "I shall succeed, there must be some way of deadening pain."[3]

The stream still flows there at Wellesley and the ducks swim gaily by, and it was to this peace and quiet that Morton again came hurrying to carry out more experiments. He started work immediately on his first subject, the family pet, a black spaniel called Nig. Fish and caterpillars were useless, and the dog was the only other subject available. According to Pereira, ether had already been used on humans, and Morton thought it safe to try on the dog. In his *Memoir on Sulphuric Ether* he describes how he inserted "the dog's head in a jar having sulphuric ether at the bottom. This was done in the presence of two persons at my house in West Needham, where I reside in the summer months. After breathing the vapour for some time the dog completely wilted in my hands. I then removed the jar. In about three minutes he aroused, yelled loudly and sprang some ten feet into a pool of water" (an exaggeration which was to be criticized severely later). But Morton was still worried about how much ether could be safely given. Every time he administered it he was afraid that he had given too much. On one occasion he really thought he had gone too far. Mrs Morton describes the scene: "One day he came running into the house in great distress (for he was always rather tender-hearted) leading the dog, which walked rather queerly, and said: 'Poor Nig, I've had him asleep a long time. I was afraid I had killed him.'"[4]

It must have been a puzzling life for his young wife. When they were just married he had a gaunt skeleton standing in a big box near the head of

56

the bed, and sometimes when she awoke in the night she found him study-ing this gruesome object. When she asked him why he behaved so strangely he just answered, "It's part of my work." When she could not understand what these ridiculous experiments had to do with his dental practice, and kept on asking him what was to become of it during all this time, he just replied, "Have patience, darling, it will all come right."[5] Mrs Morton said later, "I was only a girl of eighteen at this time, and I had not the least idea of what he was trying to do, nor would I have understood the importance of his experiments had he told me. I only knew that his clothes seemed always saturated with the smell of ether, and I did not like it."[6]

One day as Morton was just preparing to administer the ether the dog smelt it and struggled to get free. It knocked over the jar and spilt most of the ether. "I felt vexed," says Morton, "and resolved to take it myself, and did so, the next day, at my office. I inhaled from my handkerchief all the ether that was left but was not completely lost, yet thought myself so far insensible that I believed that a tooth could have been drawn with but little pain or consciousness."[7]

Leavitt, one of Morton's apprentices, tells how Morton excitedly ex-claimed, "I have got it now! I shall take my patients into the front room and extract their teeth, and then take them into the back office, put in a new set, and send them off without them knowing anything about the operation!"[8]

Apparently on the brink of success, he now became very worried in case anyone should discover his secret, and the nearer he came to success the more nervous he was that someone would find out what he was using. It was not only that he did not want anyone to snatch the prize from him, but, even more important, experience had taught him that his very living as a dentist depended on being able to offer his patients some special treat-ment which his colleagues were not able to give. So far he had done every-thing possible to keep his secret from others, and when he had asked Hayden to look after his practice for him he had begged him "not to mention what he had communicated" to him. Morton knew he was even more vulnerable because he was using only one substance, and, what is more, one which could be bought quite easily by anyone. With his supply of ether exhausted Morton became worried about continually buying ether from the same place and decided to get a large supply of ether from somewhere where nothing was known of him or his experiments. He sent one of his students over to Brewer, Stevens and Co., a well-known whole-sale house out on Washington Street, to buy a demijohn.

With this ether Morton planned to carry out some more tests. First, he asked Hayden to inhale, but he said it was no part of his duties as a locum and refused. Morton then tried his two apprentices, Spear and Leavitt. Spear had already taken part in 'ether frolics' at Lexington Academy and agreed to try. Morton gave them some to inhale separately, but to Morton's great surprise and consternation, in each case the moment they started to inhale the ether they both became so excited under its influence and yelled and thrashed about with their arms so much that they had to be held down firmly to prevent them from doing any damage or injuring themselves. Morton was astounded, for the effect on them both was so absolutely different from that on the dog Nig and on himself. He had no idea of the reason for the failure and was discouraged and disheartened. He tried to persuade the apprentices to try again, but the violent effects made them realize how dangerous it was, and this time they both backed down hastily. Although Morton offered to pay them if they would inhale again, Spear said his parents had forbidden him.

Morton was now desperate to try out the ether again on some human being and looked everywhere for someone whom he could persuade to inhale for him. He even sent his students out round the wharves to offer money to a docker, but their search was unsuccessful, for there were no volunteers in Ann-Street or Quincey Market, and mouths who he said would have readily opened to take any amount of bad rum could not be induced to take anything in the cause of medicine. But the Irish dockers had reason to be suspicious, for this was the time of the body-snatchers, when corpses were spirited away and sold for medical research. In fact, the family of St Martin, the man with a hole in his stomach, was so afraid that his body would be stolen and waited so long before bringing it to church to be buried that in the end the body stank so much that they had to leave it outside the church during the burial service. The curiosity of the medical profession was so insatiable that the 'Irish Giant' whose eight-foot-tall body had aroused so much interest was scared that his corpse would be mutilated by the anatomists, and arranged for a large sum of money to be given to boatmen to bury his body out at sea. But some-one else was prepared to pay even more, and the boatmen were given £400 —a lot of money in those days—to hand over his body to the doctors, and his skeleton now hangs in the museum at the Royal College of Surgeons in London.

Morton was very discouraged by his failure to persuade anyone to inhale for him. He would be unable to observe the results properly, but there was nothing else to be done; he must try it out again on himself. Cautiously he began inhaling, but almost immediately he was seized by the same excitement as his two assistants had been. What had happened? What could possibly have gone wrong, he asked himself. Just when it seemed he had found what he was looking for he was suddenly plunged back into failure and despair. Again he cursed his lack of real scientific education. If only he knew why the two specimens of ether had produced such very different results. If only he knew what had gone wrong. He wondered if it was the amount inhaled and whether he could devise some apparatus which would enable him to control it. But how? He must find

58

someone with expert knowledge of these subjects. Metcalf was by this time away on a trip to Europe, and he went instead to talk to Joseph Wightman, the instrument-maker.

Morton questioned him closely about different methods of inhaling. What apparatus would give the most control over the amount and rate of inhalation? What about an indiarubber bag? Would it be suitable for retaining ether? Wightman replied that ether would tend to soften the rubber and might make it leak, and when Morton asked him about oiled silk Wightman said it would probably have the same tendency. However, he insisted that he was not competent to advise him on all these questions and that Morton must consult someone more qualified, suggesting Professor Charles Jackson as the leading authority in the city. Morton's colleague Hayden also urged him to find out from Jackson the different qualities and preparations of ether with which he said all chemists were familiar.

But Morton was very loath to do this. He remembered their row, but, much more important than that, he now knew Jackson to be an unscrupulous rogue who had tried to take St Martin away from Beaumont, had fought for seven years through the highest courts in America in his attempt to claim Morse's invention, and was suggesting that he and not Schönbein had invented gun-cotton. Morton says, "I approved of the suggestion, but feared Dr Jackson might guess what I was experimenting upon, and forestall me."[9] For days he worried about what his next step should be, but by now it was August and the weather very hot. He had been overworking, and the heat again affected him so badly that he was forced to leave Boston to go to the country to recover a little.

Once again the way seemed blocked. Others might have been tempted to give up, but still he puzzled over the problem, and some weeks later he took up the challenge again: "With the autumn and the restoration of health, my ambition led me to resume my experiments." Again he went to see Hayden to ask him to continue to look after his practice. Dr Grenville Hayden was surprised by Morton's prolonged absence. He knew him to be a keen and industrious young man, previously completely devoted to his dental practice. Now here he was back in Boston, but instead of taking up his practice he asked Hayden to continue to attend to his patients. Both Morton's lawyer and his wife begged him to consider carefully what he was doing, for they were sure he was going to lose all his patients. But in spite of their protests Morton still insisted he needed more time for his experiments and asked Hayden to continue.

While he had been away Morton had been turning over in his mind what his next step ought to be, and eventually decided that there was only one thing for it: he must go to see Jackson. "I went to Dr Jackson's, therefore," he writes, "to procure a gasbag, also with the intention of ascertaining something more accurately as to the different preparations of ether, if

I should find I could do so without setting him upon the same track of experiment with myself. . . . It is enough for me to say that I felt I had made sacrifices and run risks for this object, that I believed myself to be close upon it, yet where another, with better opportunities for experimenting, availing himself of my hints and labours, might take the prize from my grasp."[10]

But although Morton knew it was his best chance of getting the technical information he needed, as he went up Beacon Hill on September 30th, 1846, past the fine old town houses with their delicately arched doorways and curved fronts, he must have still been wondering whether he was doing the right thing. He found Jackson in his laboratory, which was connected to the house by a covered way. There are two different versions of what took place there that day, Morton stating he pretended to know little about ether in case Jackson became suspicious, while Jackson claimed that Morton was in fact an ignoramus who knew nothing of ether. There seems little reason to doubt Morton's version of what happened:

> I asked Dr Jackson for his gasbag. He told me it was in his house. I went for it, and returned through the laboratory. He said, in a laughing manner, "Well, doctor, you seem to be all equipped, minus the gas." I replied, in the same manner, that perhaps there would be no need of having any gas, if the person who took it could only be made to believe there was gas in it, and alluded to the story of the man who died from being made to believe that he was bleeding to death, there being nothing but water trickling upon his leg; but I had no intention whatever of trying such a trick. He smiled, and said that was a good story, but added, in a grave manner, that I had better not attempt such an experiment, lest I should be set down as a greater humbug than Wells with his nitrous oxide gas. Seeing that here was an opportunity to open the subject, I said, in as careless a manner as I could assume, "Why cannot I give the ether gas?" He said that I could do so, and spoke again of the students taking it at Cambridge. He said the patient would be dull and stupefied, that I could do what I pleased with him, that he would not be able to help himself. Finding the subject open, I made the enquiries I wished as to the different kinds and preparations of ether. He told me something about the preparations and thinking that if he had any it would be of the purest kind, I asked him to let me see his. He did so, but remarked that it had been standing for some time, and told me that I could get some highly rectified at Burnetts.[11]

Suddenly Morton saw the reason for his failure—the first specimen of ether had come from Burnetts and was highly refined, but the large jar from Brewer Stevens had obviously been impure. In fact, according to Dr Martin Gay, who examined it later, it had more impurities than usually found in the best ether, and it was these impurities which had produced the violent results when Spear and Leavitt had behaved like lunatics. Morton waited impatiently for Jackson to finish, but it seemed as if he was never going to stop. Jackson was always most talkative, with a steady stream of anecdotes showing how clever he was and what fine friends he had. Morton was by now anxious only to escape. He desperately wanted to try inhaling again with the pure ether, and he could hardly bear to stand there while Jackson rambled on. At last he was prepared to let him go, but as Morton moved towards the door Jackson followed him, still talking. He suggested using some other apparatus than a gasbag, and handed Morton a flask with a glass tube in it.

With the words "pure, rectified ether" ringing in his ears Morton rushed straight round to Burnetts. He could hardly contain his excitement as he ordered various drugs, and then, casually, as if the matter was of little importance, he asked for a small flask of rectified ether to be added to his order. He raced back to his office next door in Tremont Row, and, having given orders that he was on no account to be disturbed, he locked himself in, sat down in his dental chair with his watch in his hand, and started immediately to inhale. He reported the experience later to the Paris Academy of Arts and Sciences:

> Taking the tube and flask, I shut myself up in a room, seated myself in the operating chair, and commenced inhaling. I found the ether so strong that it partially suffocated me, but produced no decided effect. I then saturated my handkerchief and inhaled from that. I looked at my watch and soon lost consciousness. As I recovered, I felt a numbness in my limbs, with a sensation like a nightmare, and would have given the world for someone to come and arouse me. I thought for a moment I should die in that state, and the world would only pity or ridicule my folly. At length I felt a slight tingling of the blood in the end of my third finger, and made an effort to touch it with my thumb, but without success. At a second effort I touched it, but there seemed to be no sensation. I gradually raised my arm and pinched my thigh, but I could see that sensation was imperfect. I attempted to rise from my chair, but fell back. Gradually I regained power over my limbs and full consciousness. I immediately looked at my watch, and found that I had been insensible between seven and eight minutes. I am firmly convinced that at that time a tooth could have been drawn without feeling of pain or consciousness.[12]

As soon as Morton had recovered sufficiently he unlocked the door and rushed into the workshop shouting "Eureka! Eureka!" dancing around the room, and clapping his assistants on the back. Mrs Morton tells how:

> That night he came home late, in a great state of excitement, but so happy that he could scarcely calm himself to tell me what had occurred; and I, too, became so excited that I could scarcely wait to hear. At last he told me of the experiment upon himself, and I grew sick at heart as the thought came to me that he might have died there alone. He went on to say that he was resolved not to sleep that night until he had repeated the experiment.[13]

It was already late and the surgery was closed, but Morton felt absolutely certain someone was going to turn up and went back to his office to wait. He was quite right, for, says Mrs Morton, late that evening:

there came a faint ring at the bell.

It was long past the hour for patients, but there stood a man with his face all bandaged and evidently suffering acute pain. And strangest of all were his words.

"Doctor," he said, "I have the most frightful toothache, and my mouth is so sore I am afraid to have the tooth drawn. Can't you mesmerize me?"

The doctor could almost have shouted with delight, but, preserving his self-possession, he brought the man into his office and told him he could do something better than mesmerize him. Then he explained his purpose of administering the ether, and the man eagerly consented. Without delay my husband saturated a handkerchief with ether, and held it over the man's face, for him to inhale the fumes. The assistant, Dr Hayden, who held the lamp, trembled visibly when Dr Morton introduced the forceps into the mouth of the man and prepared to pull the tooth. Then came the strain, the wrench, and the tooth was out, but the patient made neither sign nor sound; he was quite unconscious.

Dr Morton was overjoyed at the result. Then, as the man continued to make no movement, he grew alarmed, and it flashed through his mind that perhaps he had killed his patient. Snatching up a glass of water, he emptied it full into the face of the unconscious man, who presently opened his eyes and looked about him in a bewildered way.

"Are you ready now to have the tooth out?" asked the doctor.

"I am ready," said the man.

"Well, it is out now," said the doctor, pointing to the tooth lying on the floor.

"No!" cried the man in greatest amazement, springing from the chair, and, being a good Methodist, shouting "Glory! Hallelujah!"[14]

Morton too must have offered up a prayer as he saw the patient lying apparently dead in the chair and knowing he stood to be accused of manslaughter. The man, Eben Frost, gave his own account, countersigned by Hayden:

This is to certify that I applied to Dr Morton at nine o'clock this evening (September 30, 1846), suffering under the most violent toothache; that Dr Morton took out his pocket handkerchief, saturated it with a preparation of his, from which I breathed for about half a minute, and then was lost in sleep. In an instant more I awoke and saw my tooth lying upon the floor. I did not experience the slightest pain whatever. I remained twenty minutes in his office afterward, and felt no unpleasant effects from the operation.[15]

Morton could now offer his patients painless extractions, and he lost no time in making capital out of it. Advertising was already a well-accepted

62

part of American life, even for dentists. The newspapers were full of their advertisements promising miraculous treatments and quick cures, and Morton went directly to see A. G. Tenney, a reporter on the Boston *Daily Journal*, to get him to write a report on the extraction of Frost's tooth, but keeping the contents of his preparation secret. He had to agree first to take advertising space, and the notice appeared in the *Daily Journal* of October 1st:

> Last evening, as we were informed by a gentleman who witnessed the operation, an ulcerated tooth was extracted from the mouth of an individual without giving him the slightest pain. He was put into a kind of sleep, by inhaling a preparation, the effects of which lasted for about three-quarters of a minute, just long enough to extract the tooth.

Morton worked hard exploiting his new painless extractions, for, like everyone else in this new and burgeoning country, he was determined to make his fortune. America had been colonized by Puritans, but men have never had much difficulty in finding reasons for their desires, and they argued that as hard work was a moral duty for all Puritans, and since hard work resulted in wealth, wealth itself must therefore represent attention to duty and its acquisition something laudable. The Puritan conscience thus became the driving force towards economic advance, and money-making became sanctified. This view was supported also by the wave of new immigrants pouring into America, for where previously men had fled from religious persecution, now the new immigrants were flooding in with one aim—to make for themselves and their families a better life than the harsh and often poverty-stricken one they had left behind. They took to the Utilitarian philosophy of their adopted country and added their voices to the clamour for material wealth. "Money", wrote Emerson, "is, in its effects and laws, as beautiful as roses. Property keeps the account of the world and is always moral. The property will be found where labour, the wisdom and the virtue have been."[16]

Morton was no different to the rest, and his one aim after painlessly removing Frost's tooth was to try to cash in on his discovery. The very next day, October 1st, he went to see Richard Eddy, who acted as the Commissioner of Patents in Boston, to apply for a patent. Eddy was not sure if the preparation could be patented or not, but promised to find out.

While Morton was waiting for a decision he did all he could to publicize his painless extraction and to exploit his secret preparation. He went to see Jackson to ask him for a testimonial like the one he had given Wells for his dental solder, but although Morton showed him the statements signed by Frost, Hayden, and Tenney, Jackson would have nothing to do with it. Morton says he asked him to "give me a certificate that it [his preparation] was harmless in its effect. This he positively refused to do." Jackson seemed not to know much about the subject or what Morton was doing.

63

Much later he asked Francis Whitman, Morton's brother-in-law, how they were getting on with the gas, and when Whitman replied that they were getting along "first rate" Jackson commented that although he knew of ether's effects when used by students, he did not know how it would work in pulling teeth. He continued to be sceptical about the results Morton was achieving, and is reported to have said to someone, "People will not believe in the insensibility to pain in the case of a mere tooth, since it is very common for patients to say it did not hurt them when the twitch is very sudden and the operation skilfully performed."[17]

Even when Morton's treatment began to become popular Jackson still went round saying it was dangerous. He told Caleb Eddy, the Commissioner of Patents' father, that Morton was a reckless, daredevil fellow and that he would kill somebody yet. He told another that "it should be used with greatest care; and that it would be very likely to injure the brain if repeated . . . and if it were, asphyxia, coma, or even death itself, might ensue".[18] He was clearly not anxious to have anything to do with such a foolhardy venture, and when Dr Gould, a friend of Morton's, remarked to him that the new treatment looked like being a success Jackson replied, "Well, let him get on with it; I don't care what he does with it, if he don't bring my name in with it."[19] But although Jackson and many of his professional colleagues refused to accept Morton's claims, patients were flocking to see him, and his surgery was constantly crowded. It seemed that everyone in Boston wanted to come and try the new treatment for themselves, and all those who had been unable to pluck up courage now came rushing to him to have their teeth removed painlessly.

But it was not all easy going. Morton still had difficulty in administering the ether, and particularly in controlling the amount inhaled. When he gave it to one woman it produced no other effect than drowsiness, and when he used the apparatus he had devised she nearly suffocated. He tried hard to get consistent results and experimented with several different types of apparatus—an indiarubber bag to hold the ether, near the neck of which he cut a small hole in the shape of a whistle for the admission of atmospheric air; a sponge soaked with ether inside a glass globe or rubber bag from which the patient inhaled; and with Wightman he devised a glass globe, all of them designed so that the patient breathed a mixture of ether fumes and air. He and Wightman spent a great deal of time and trouble devising the apparatus, but when he used their globe on one patient Morton described how "she seemed to be in an unnatural state, but continued talking, and refused to have the tooth extracted. I made her some trifling offer, to which she assented, and drew the tooth, without any indication of pain on her part, not a muscle moving."[20] Morton noted that her pulse was 90, her face much flushed, and after she came round she was excessively drowsy for a long time afterwards. When he gave Miss L. his preparation the effect was "rather alarming. She sprang up from the chair,

64

leaped into the air, screamed, and was held down with difficulty."[21] When she came to she was unconscious of what had happened, but was willing for him to administer the ether again, which he did with success.

Morton was still constantly being made aware of the great dangers. When he administered the preparation to a boy it produced "no other effect than sickness, with vomiting, and the boy was taken home in a coach, and pronounced by a physician to be poisoned. His friends were excited, and threatened proceedings against me."[22] Rumours began to circulate round the town about people almost dying in the chair and only just being saved by timely action. Other dentists became jealous too when they saw their patients flocking to Morton, and started a movement to prevent him continuing with his new treatment. Soon they were joined by conservative members of the medical profession who had seen mesmerism and other false claims come and go and were convinced that a dentist with no qualifications like Morton could not possibly have discovered something which for centuries had eluded all the greatest scientists.

Morton was too busy perfecting his method to bother much about the rumours and criticisms. He worked day and night trying out all sorts of apparatus and noting carefully the reactions of each patient, for sometimes very little ether was needed to make a patient unconscious, while for others the inhaling had to be prolonged. Morton had noticed too that the mental attitude of the patient had an effect on the results achieved and used his first patient, Eben Frost, to allay the fears of other patients. Frost had left his job as a music teacher and now spent all his time helping Morton and recommending his treatment.

He was also constantly at Morton's side to act as a witness to secure recognition for his discovery in medical circles, for although Morton had set out originally to find something which would save his patients pain during the extraction of teeth, it did not take long for him to realize that his discovery had much more far-reaching possibilities. He believed it might be possible to extend its use to surgical operations, and his work was now devoted to saving humanity that even more terrifying pain.

NOTES TO CHAPTER VI

1. Sarah J. Hale, *Godey's Lady's Book.*
2. *McClure's Magazine*, September 1896.
3. *Ibid.*
4. *Ibid.*
5. *Ibid.*
6. *Ibid.*
7. W. Morton, *Memoir on Sulphuric Ether.*
8. *Littell's Living Age,* 1848.
9. Morton, *op. cit.*
10. *Ibid.*

E

11. Nathan Rice, *Trials of a Public Benefactor.*
12. Morton, *op. cit.*
13. *McClure's Magazine,* September 1896.
14. *Ibid.*
15. Nathan Rice, *op. cit.*
16. R. W. Emerson, *Complete Works.*
17. Nathan Rice, *op. cit.*
18. *Ibid.*
19. *Ibid.*
20. *Ibid.*
21. *Ibid.*
22. *Ibid.*

CHAPTER

VII

WHEN Morton began his work medicine was still very primitive. Doctors prescribed bleeding and sweating as a cure for everything, even advocating bleeding until four-fifths of the blood had been drawn away. No wonder William Cobbett said, "Blood, blood, still they cry more blood!" Surgical operations were performed under the most ghastly conditions, and the surgeon was little more than a skilled butcher, enormously strong and aided not by pretty, comforting nurses, but by great brutes whose job it was to hold down the screaming patient. The eighteenth-century anatomist John Hunter described the surgeon as "a savage armed with a knife", and an operation "a humiliating spectacle of the futility of science". Some doctors vomited when they left the operating theatre. Some went with two bottles of strong alcoholic liquor—one for themselves and one for the patient. Some tried opium in various forms. Some administered nicotine, by inserting a cigar into the patient's rectum or having smoke puffed into it. But alcohol, nicotine, opium, nothing could assuage the terrible agony of the surgeon's knife. "Not poppy, nor mandragora, nor all the drowsy syrups of the world"[1] could save them that. Once the operation started even the bravest screamed and struggled to be free of the agonizing pain.

Only the simplest operations could be performed or the patient died on the operating table from the pain and shock. Any delay resulted in the death of the patient from heart-failure, and the best surgeons were those who worked quickest. William Cheselden, the friend of Alexander Pope, could cut out a stone in the bladder in fifty-four seconds. Lagenbeck, the chief surgeon of the Hanoverian Army, was said to perform an amputation at the shoulder-joint in the time needed to take a pinch of snuff. Liston, the Scottish surgeon, famous for the speed of his operations, could complete an amputation, including ligatures, in twenty-nine seconds. It is difficult to appreciate their desperate speed when operations can now last many hours. It is even more difficult to imagine the terrifying agonies of operations performed before Morton made his discovery. A writer in Morton's time described an operation for a dislocated hip-joint:

A pulley is attached to the affected limb, while the body, trussed up by appropriate bands, is fastened to another; now several powerful, muscular assistants seize the ropes, and with a careful, steady drawing, tighten the cords. Soon the tension makes itself felt, and as the stubborn muscles stretch and yield to the strain, one can almost imagine that he hears the crack of parting sinews. Big drops of perspiration, started by the excess of agony, bestrew the patient's forehead, sharp screams burst from him in peal after peal—all his struggles to free himself and escape the horrid torture, are valueless, for he is in the powerful hands of men then as inexorable as death. . . . Stronger comes the pull, more force is added to the ropes, the tugs, cruel and unyielding, seem as if they would burst the tendons where they stand out like whipcords. At last the agony becomes too great for human endurance, and with a wild, despairing yell, the suffering patient relapses into unconsciousness. . . . The surgeon avails himself of this opportunity and . . . seizing the limb by a dexterous twist snaps the head of the bone into its socket. The operation is done, and the poor prostrated, bruised sufferer can be removed to his pallet to recover from the fearful results of the operation as best he can.[2]

In fact, few patients ever did recover from surgery, and doctors operated only when everything else had failed. They dared not tell the patient of the dangers, and once when someone asked the great surgeon Liston whether the amputation of his leg was going to hurt, Liston replied encouragingly, "No more than having a tooth out." "Then I'll have it done tomorrow (Saturday)," said the man, "then I shall be all right on Sunday." "Very well, so be it!"[3] answered Liston. It seems another world, and, indeed, it was. Streets were piled high with refuse, dead bodies lay one upon the other in crypts and cellars, hospitals were filthy. Although it was a time of great elegance, in even the highest circles standards of hygiene were abysmally low. Indoor sanitation was almost unknown, and in the elegant furniture of Hepplewhite's time, while one part of the sideboard contained cutlery and drinking water, the other pedestal contained a pot cupboard in which the gentlemen urinated after dinner. In such a society it is not surprising that the hospitals were equally unhygienic. Operating theatres were filthy, had no ventilation, no heating, and no running water. The operating table was a dirty wooden slab. Surgeons wore not a shining white antiseptic gown, but an old, blood-stained frockcoat.

The filth and pain are horrifying, but were then regarded as absolutely

68

inevitable. All the greatest scientific authorities agreed that there was no way of preventing pain. All Morton's teachers constantly told him that he must accept pain as part of the normal reaction of the human body. They insisted that for a mere student to attempt to question such immutable scientific laws was not only foolhardy but would surely lead to a prosecution for manslaughter. But Morton refused to accept their edicts. He had dedicated his life to finding a pain-killer, and once more he set to work and once again, to the dismay of his wife and friends, left his practice in the hands of Dr Hayden and his assistants. No one could understand Morton at all. He had set out originally to find a method of extracting and crowning teeth painlessly, and had succeeded beyond all his wildest expectations. Patients were flocking to his surgery for his new treatment, and he could have relaxed and just enjoyed being the most popular dentist in town. But had he done so painless surgery would have been indefinitely delayed, and patients would have continued to suffer their terrible agonies.

So again he gave up everything to experiment, for, although he now believed it would be possible to extend the use of ether inhalation to surgery, he still had to discover how to regulate the artificial sleep and strengthen and prolong it. Within a matter of days he felt ready to talk to doctors and to ask for a proper trial for his discovery. But it was difficult. Wherever he went he met with stern resistance from the medical profession. It might be supposed that surgeons would have snatched at a chance to save their patients pain and to have the opportunity of operating on their patients calmly and peacefully. But when Morton canvassed the doctors he met with rebuffs. Drugs, herbs, mesmerism, somnambulism, operating on frozen limbs, even such foolhardy methods as pressing on patients' carotid arteries, nearly throttling them in an effort to deprive their brains of fresh blood—and then, only a year before, Wells's own ridiculous experiment with laughing gas—all made them reluctant to consider such a revolutionary idea. How could they treat seriously such a dangerous proposition put forward by a mere dentist. Were they to believe that he had achieved what the greatest scientific minds had so far failed to do?

Their scepticism was infuriating to Morton, but fortunately there was a young surgeon in Boston whose mind was also attuned to the new scientific age, and when he saw Morton's announcement in the papers he asked if he could come to watch him using his new treatment. H. J. Bigelow, son of the great Boston physician Dr Jacob Bigelow, had graduated from Harvard when only fifteen. He had studied medicine in America and Europe and had come back with a taste for new things. He brought a cabriolet from France, and the black horse with its scarlet leather monogrammed harness and his own French clothes and manners startled the sober puritanical New England society. But in spite of these he was a first-class surgeon; at twenty-six he won the Boyleston Prize with his *Manual of Orthopaedic Surgery*, and was soon appointed to be visiting surgeon to the Massachusetts General Hospital.

Quick to appreciate innovations, he took to Morton immediately, recognizing the importance of his discovery, and supporting him enthusiastically throughout. He watched Morton and made notes on the cases, and afterwards spoke highly about him to Dr Warren, the same great Boston surgeon who had presided when Wells had made such a fool of himself. Morton also called on Warren's son, Mason, and demonstrated his new treatment. John Collins Warren was an awe-inspiring man of sixty-eight, of tremendous fame and authority, a stern Puritan and a temperance man, and the most eminent surgeon in all New England. He had studied at Harvard, abroad in Paris, Edinburgh, and in London at Guy's Hospital under the great Sir Astley Cooper. He had completely revolutionized medical education in America and had started the *New England Journal of Medicine and Surgery*. He was the first surgeon in America to operate for a strangulated hernia and was an authority on tumours. He was altogether a formidable man, and Morton must have been quaking in his shoes when he went to see him. But Warren listened to Morton sympathetically. He told Morton that he had always hoped to find something to alleviate the pain of surgical operations and that he had in fact experimented himself with various substances, but with the most unsatisfactory results. He said also that he realized the immensity of the task and would do everything in his power to help.

In between campaigning Morton was busy perfecting his method of administering the ether. He worked hard on his experiments, but each day he hoped and waited anxiously for news from Warren. On Wednesday, October 14th, the letter came. Dr C. F. Heywood, house surgeon at the Massachusetts General Hospital, wrote:

DEAR SIR,
I write at the request of Dr John Collins Warren to invite you to be present Friday Morning, October 16, at ten o'clock at the hospital to administer to a patient who is then to be operated upon, the preparation you have invented to diminish the sensibility to pain.[4]

Warren's son said that the day before the letter was written a young printer, Gilbert Abbott, was brought into the operating room of the hospital. As Warren prepared for the operation he said suddenly, "I now remember that I have made a promise to Mr Morton to give him an opportunity to try out a new remedy for preventing pain in surgical operations." He then explained to the patient that this preparation might well save him much of the pain he was bound to suffer and asked whether he would be willing to submit himself to a test of it, in spite of the risks which might be involved. Absolutely terrified of having an operation, Abbott

70

naturally jumped at the chance of anything which could possibly save him pain.

So the time had come for Morton to demonstrate his discovery to the world, but still he was worried about the apparatus. In the brief fortnight since he had made his first extraction under ether he had already introduced several refinements, both to his apparatus and to his method of administering the ether. In his *Memoir* he says:

> When the time drew near for the experiment at the hospital, I became exceedingly anxious, and gave all my time, day and night, hardly sleeping or eating, to the contriving of my apparatus, and general investigation of the subject. I called on Dr Gould, a physician who has paid much attention to chemistry and told him my anxieties. He sympathized with me, gave me his attention and we sat up nearly all night making sketches of apparatus; he first suggesting to me an antidote in case of unfavourable effects, and the valvular system, instead of the one I used.

Joseph Wightman, the instrument-maker, relates how Morton called one afternoon "in a great hurry" to beg his help in getting the apparatus ready for the trial:

> He appeared very much excited, and although from pressure of other engagements it was very inconvenient for me, yet I consented to arrange a temporary apparatus under these circumstances. This was composed of a quart tubulated globe receiver, having a cork fitted into it instead of a glass stopper, through which cork a pipette or dropping tube was inserted to supply the ether as it was evaporated. I then cut several large grooves around the cork to admit the air freely into the globe, to mix with the vapour, and delivered it to Dr Morton.[5]

Morton was so worried that he also asked Chamberlain, another technician, to make him an inhaler, and this was the one he actually used. It was a two-necked glass globe, one neck permitting the free inflow of air. The other opening was fitted with a wooden mouthpiece through which the patient breathed in air across the surface of the ether in the bottom of the jar, so charging the air with ether vapour. The amount of fumes and air that the patient breathed was regulated by a tap on the mouthpiece.

Morton was now even more worried about the possible dangers. He had used ether so far only in dentistry, and although he had worked at it until he considered his method foolproof, he knew that the effects of ether were unpredictable. All the authorities agreed that it was highly dangerous: Faraday, in the *Quarterly Journal of Science and the Arts*, said, "By the incautious breathing of ether vapour a man was thrown into a lethargic condition which, with a few interruptions, lasted for 30 hours." Pereira described a case in which stupefaction ensued where "for many days the pulse was so much lowered that considerable fears were entertained for the safety of the patient. In another one, an apoplectic condition, which continued for some hours was produced."

71

Morton was terrified that something might go wrong. If he gave too little ether the patient would scream and struggle and he would be disgraced and his preparation abandoned. If he gave too much the patient would die and he would be held responsible for his death. It was a situation which would have daunted most people, but, displaying that supremely great courage which marks the world's greatest discoverers, Morton decided to go through with the test. Mrs Morton describes her own fears:

> The night before the operation my husband worked until one or two o'clock in the morning upon his inhaler. I assisted him, nearly beside myself with anxiety, for the strongest influences had been brought to bear upon me to dissuade him from making this attempt. I had been told that one of two things was sure to happen: either the test would fail and my husband would be ruined by the world's ridicule, or he would kill the patient and be tried for manslaughter. Thus I was drawn in two ways; for while I had unbounded confidence in my husband, it did not seem possible that so young a man [he was only twenty-seven years old at this time] could be wiser than the learned and scientific men before whom he proposed to make his demonstration.[6]

It was these dangers which kept going through and through Morton's head as he tried to snatch some rest in the few hours of the night which still remained. He got up early to rush off to collect the new inhaler from Chamberlain. It was supposed to be ready by eight o'clock, but when Morton got there Chamberlain was still working on it. Some last changes had been needed, but as the minutes ticked by and the time for the operation got nearer and nearer Morton became more and more nervous and impatient. Continually he begged Chamberlain to hurry with his work, until at last, afraid he was going to be too late, he snatched the instrument from the man's hands and dashed off for the hospital.

In his pocket he carried a bottle of ether flavoured with some aromatic, oil of oranges, perhaps, and opium, to prevent people recognizing the smell and guessing what his preparation contained. Frost accompanied him as usual to vouch for the new treatment, and as Morton ran on full pelt down Cambridge Street, his head bent, his cloak billowing out around him, Frost followed puffing behind. Through Blossom and Fruit Street they ran, towards the hospital building, its huge Bulfinch dome dominating the Charles River from where patients were brought by boat and carried straight into the hospital. As they dashed breathlessly on Morton continued to be tormented about the consequences of what he was about to do, and barely managed to keep his nerve. Suppose the patient should be a drunk and the ether have no effect, suppose it be a swooning young girl who refused to inhale properly, suppose the patient screamed and struggled so much that the surgeons were obliged to interfere and had to ask him to retire, suppose . . . suppose . . . so many fearful thoughts kept

72

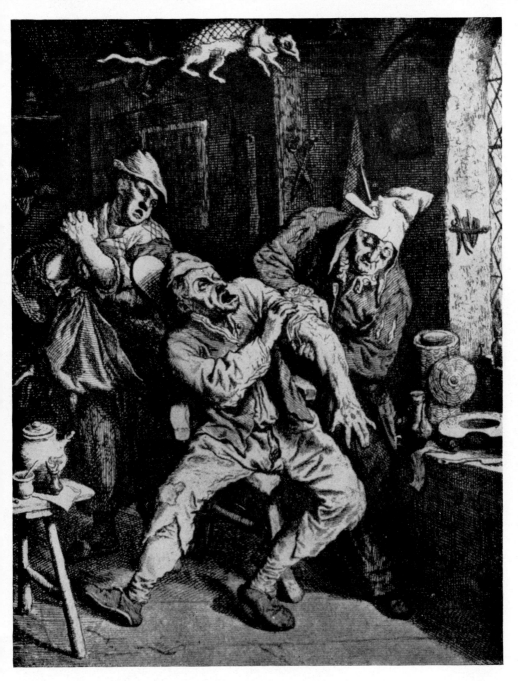

A barber-surgeon operating

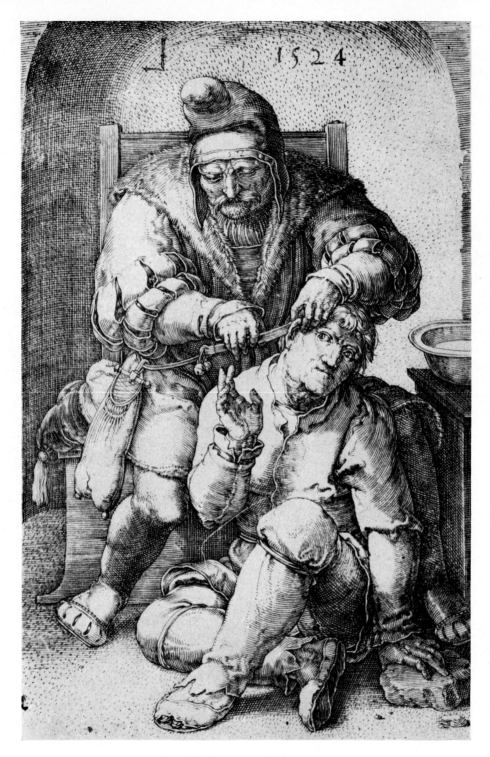

Operation for a mastoid in 1524

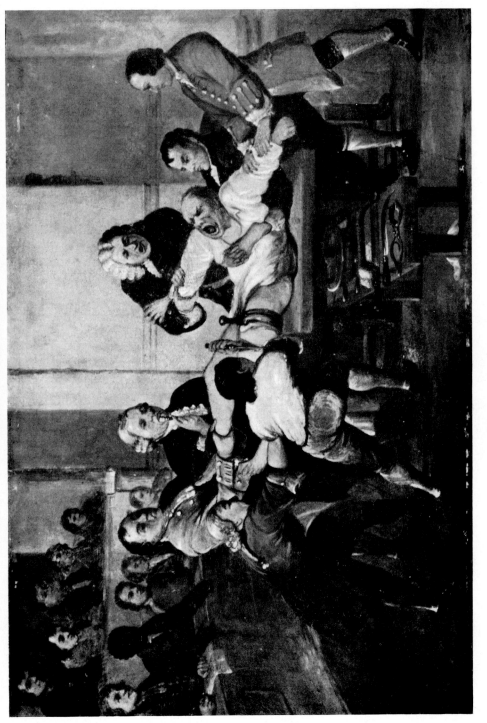

Amputation of a leg at the thigh

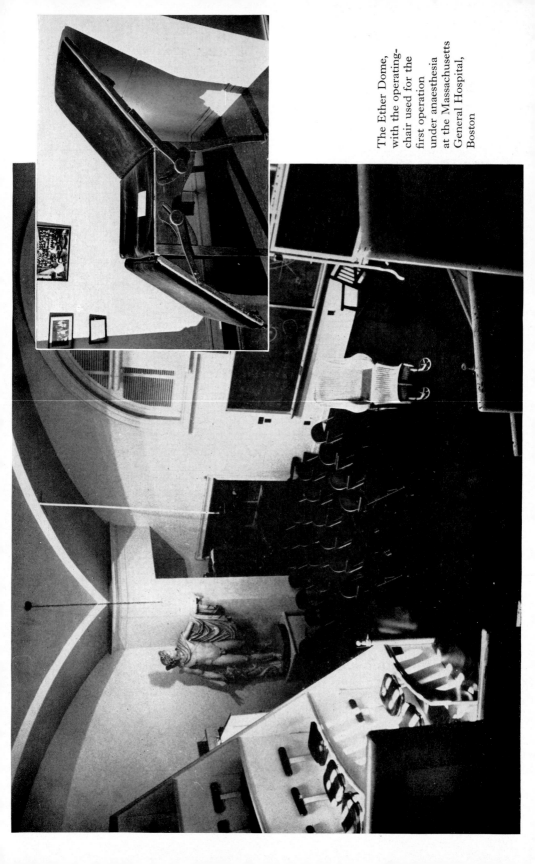

The Ether Dome, with the operating-chair used for the first operation under anaesthesia at the Massachusetts General Hospital, Boston flooding into his mind as they ran on, until, hardly pausing at the entrance to the great granite building, they leapt up the steps to the portico, through its eight grand Ionic columns, and on up the stairs towards the operating theatre.

The Ether Dome, as it is now called, is still preserved high up in the old building immediately beneath the central dome, and leading up to it are the simple granite staircases with their curved wooden handrails and old Colonial lanterns. Inside is a small amphitheatre with rows of seats ranged in ascending ranks up to the ceiling of the dome. In the corners, standing upright in their painted coffins, are the two Egyption mummies brought all the way from Thebes, one with its head unwrapped from linen bindings to reveal a blackened, shrunken face. It must have been a gruesome sight for a patient to face this horrifying corpse beside him, and in Morton's day, too, along one side were large cases full of long rows of glittering knives, saws, and other surgical appliances, carefully arranged in order. In various parts of the room were tables and chairs of different patterns; hooks, rings, and pulleys were inserted into the wall, and everywhere something met the eye which had been obviously designed for some specific and terrible purpose.

The operating theatre was now full of eminent medical men and crowded out with students. They had been assembled for some time, and, drawn there by the reports of Morton's marvellous new preparation, were almost all the Boston surgeons. Heading them was the great Dr John C. Warren himself, senior surgeon at the hospital, one of its founders, and its chief for thirty years. Warren was a tall, thin man, with deeply lined features and a large hooked nose. As he stood beside the operating chair he looked a forbidding figure, staring out haughtily through bright, piercing eyes over the assembled audience. George Hayward, his assistant, was there beside him, tall, blond, commanding, with a cold, fixed expression, and with them Jacob Bigelow, said to be one of the wisest and greatest men ever to adorn the profession, and his already famous young surgeon son, Henry J. Bigelow, "perhaps," said Mrs Morton, "the only man present who had faith in Morton." Seated in front were S. D. Townsend, Samuel Parkman, J. G. Pearson, Heywood, Gould, and Wellington, and many others of equal fame and distinction. Behind them the seats were crowded with medical students.

It was now ten o'clock, the time set for the operation and the patient, Gilbert Abbott, had been brought in and placed on the operating couch. He was a young man of twenty who was to have a tumour removed from under his jaw. Dressed in breeches with a crumpled shirt open at the neck, he lay there deathly white, desperately frightened of what was to come. Dr Warren stepped forwards and made an announcement. In his high-pitched but brusquely commanding voice he told them that a test of some preparation was to be carried out by Morton for which the "astonishing claim had been made that it would render the person operated upon free from pain. . . . I have always regarded this condition as an important desideratum in operative surgery, as you are well aware, so I decided to let him try the experiment."[7]

As the hands of the clock started past ten the distinguished gathering, already very sceptical of the reports they had heard, began to voice their doubts about the whole affair and to stir restlessly in their seats. The minutes ticked by. The stillness was oppressive. Five minutes passed, then ten, and still there was no sign of Morton. Dr Warren took out his watch from his pocket and checked the time against it. It was almost a quarter past ten. The assembled crowd began to fidget, and in spite of Dr Warren's commanding presence their whispered conversations became louder as they declared that Morton was obviously too scared to show his face after suggesting such a ridiculous experiment. Amid this tense atmosphere Warren stood nervously smoothing his coat-tails, continually glancing angrily towards the door. Finally, with a last look at the time, he resolutely picked up the surgical knife and, looking at the packed benches with a sarcastic smile on his face, said, "As Dr Morton has not arrived, I presume he is otherwise engaged." There was a burst of derisive laughter from the crowded room as the attendants swiftly strapped down the patient and Dr Warren sat down to his patient to operate.

Just at that moment the door was flung open and Morton rushed in breathlessly. He had his inhaler in his hand and was followed by a flustered Frost, puffing and blowing after him. Deeply embarrassed, Morton began to stammer an apology for being so late and to give the reason for it when Warren cut him sternly short. "Well, sir, your patient is ready." Taking the man by the hand, Morton spoke a few encouraging words to him, assuring him that he would partially relieve, if not entirely prevent, the pain of the operation. Pointing to Frost, Morton told him that this was a man who had taken ether and would testify to its success. "Are you afraid?" Morton asked. "No," replied the man; "I feel confident, and will do precisely what you tell me."[8]

Mrs Morton takes up the story: "Without delay, and with a coolness and self-possession in strong contrast with the general nervous tension of the assembly," Morton began to administer his preparation. Should he succeed it would be the first time in the world's history that the alleviation of pain in a surgical operation had ever been publicly demonstrated. But the faces of the expectant crowd were no pleasant or reassuring picture, for on each one there was an expression of plain incredulity, if not open hostility. Morton was undeterred. "Pouring the liquid into the inhaler," says Mrs Morton, "he lifted the latter to the patient's nostrils, and held it there for some minutes, allowing the man to breathe the fumes. Then, looking into his face intently, and feeling the pulse, he turned to Dr Warren, who stood near with his surgeon's knife behind him, and said in

74

a quiet tone that sounded plainly through the silence: 'Your patient is ready, doctor.' "[9]

Morton had been concentrating hard on his task, but even he could not have failed to notice that the rustling from the audience as they strained to get a better view had been succeeded by the most breathless silence, and as he turned to Dr Warren he saw that the looks of incredulity and contempt had given place to expressions of astonishment.

Mrs Morton goes on:

Then in all parts of the amphitheatre there came a quick catching of breath, followed by a silence almost deathlike, as Dr Warren stepped forward and prepared to operate. The sheet was thrown back, exposing the portion of the body from which a tumour was to be removed, an operation exceedingly painful under ordinary conditions, although neither very difficult nor very dangerous. The patient lay silent, with eyes closed as if in sleep; but everyone present fully expected to hear a shriek of agony ring out as the knife struck down into the sensitive nerves. But the stroke came with no accompanying cry. Then another and another, and still the patient lay silent, sleeping while the blood from the severed artery spurted forth. The surgeon was doing his work, and the patient was free from pain, so it seemed at least; and all in wonder strained their eyes and bent forward, following eagerly every step in the operation.[10]

The distinguished doctors in front leaned over or knelt down on the board floor so that those behind might have a better view. All eyes were riveted upon this extraordinary scene, while everyone was still and immovable as the skeletons and mummies in the cases behind them. The operation advanced quickly and easily to its finish. The tumour was taken away, the arteries fastened with ligatures, the gaping wound sewn up and dressed and bandaged. It was all over in half an hour, and during all that time not a cry or groan had come from the patient. Morton aroused him and said, "Did you feel any pain?" "No," replied the man. Dr Warren then turned to the company and said quietly and impressively, "Gentlemen, this is no humbug!"[11]

For a moment the spectators sat still in silent awe. Then, suddenly, the tension was broken, and they surged forward to congratulate Morton and to shower him with their questions. They all wanted to examine the patient and to ask again his reactions. Did he really feel nothing? "I have experienced no pain," he told them, "but only a sensation like that of scraping the part with a blunt instrument."[12] Now there could be no doubt that Morton's discovery was a great and sensational success. After years of grinding work and laborious experiment he had finally discovered an effective pain-killer. Where through the ages all the great medical and scientific minds of the world had failed, Morton had succeeded beyond his utmost expectations. Now, in one of the most famous hospitals in all

America, eminent surgeons crowded round to shake him by the hand and hastened to congratulate him on his phenomenal success. It was indeed a proud moment for the humble, uneducated dentist.

Here was the practicability of what he had imagined completely and satisfactorily proved to all the world; and as he stood there full of pride at his great success, his brain giddy with excitement, he was the centre of attraction of all that great and distinguished company. For the first time in the history of the world it had been publicly demonstrated that a surgical operation could be accomplished without the screams and struggles which had always accompanied the agonies of the knife. For the first time in the history of the world Morton appeared to have conquered pain. It seemed as if his work was finished and his fame and success assured—but in reality the struggle of his life had only just begun.

NOTES TO CHAPTER VII

1. *Othello.*
2. Nathan Rice, *Trials of a Public Benefactor.*
3. *American Journal of Surgery*, 29 (Anaesthesia Supplement), 1951.
4. Nathan Rice, *op. cit.*
5. *Ibid.*
6. *McClure's Magazine,* September 1896.
7. Nathan Rice, *op. cit.*
8. *Ibid.*
9. *McClure's Magazine,* September 1896.
10. *Ibid.*
11. *Ibid.*
12. *Nathan Rice, op. cit.*

CHAPTER

VIII

WHEN Morton changed surgical operations from screaming "humiliating spectacles" he changed the life of the world. He also catastrophically changed his own. Mrs Morton tells of his return from the operation on that historic day:

I saw nothing of him for twelve hours, which were hours of mortal anxiety. How they dragged along as I sat at the window, expecting every moment some messenger to tell me that the patient had died under the ether and that the doctor would be held responsible! Two o'clock came, three o'clock, and it was not until nearly four that Dr Morton walked in, with his usual genial face so sad that I felt failure must have come. He took me in his arms, almost fainting as I was, and said tenderly: "Well, dear, I succeeded!"

In spite of these words, his gloom of manner and evident depression made it impossible for me to believe the good news. It seemed as if he should have been so highly elated at having accomplished one of the most splendid achievements of the century, and yet there he was, sick at heart, crushed down, one would have said, by a load of discouragement. This was due not only to bodily fatigue and the reaction after his great efforts, but to an intuitive perception of the troubles in store for him. It is literally true that Dr Morton never was the same man after that day; his whole life was embittered through this priceless boon he had conferred upon the human race.[1]

At first all went well for Morton. The following day he administered his new preparation and Dr George Hayward, Warren's assistant, removed a tumour from a woman's arm. The "artificial sleep" was successfully induced, and the patient again appeared to be unaware of the pain. But in spite of his great success, Morton realized that there was still much more to be done to perfect his method of painless surgery. In the first flush of

77

excitement for the new discovery the eyewitness accounts stated that the patients had shown no signs of pain, but actually, as Bigelow pointed out in the precise scientific statement which he gave three weeks later before the Boston Society of Medical Improvement, there were already indications of considerable problems.

In the first operation, on Abbott on October 16th, "the patient muttered, as in a semi-conscious state, and afterwards stated that the pain was considerable, though mitigated".[2] In the second operation to remove a tumour the patient "betrayed marks of uneasiness".[3] Bigelow recorded also that Morton had trouble even in his dental operations: in some cases it had been difficult to get the patients to inhale the gas at all, as they coughed so much, while in others his preparation appeared to have no effect even when inhaling had been continued for half an hour; in one case a woman became so excited during inhalation that she had to be held down in the chair, while some patients continued to be unconscious for an hour after inhalation; in very young children there was nausea and vomiting; in some cases the patient's pulse rose to as high as 144.

Even in the later operations there was considerable anxiety about the patient's condition, and Bigelow described a protracted inhalation which had been continued for thirty-five minutes or so when the pulse suddenly dropped from 120 to 96, the breathing became slow, the hands deathly cold, and the patient insensible. The doctors became worried, tried to stimulate the breathing and circulation, and treated the patient as they did at that time for poisoning—applying cold effusions to his head, syringing his ears, and administering ammonia by smell, and internally as well. The symptoms remained for fifteen minutes, and they had to bring the patient round by making him move his limbs and walking him up and down for half an hour. If he had not already had a haemorrhage from the nose they would have bled him as well. Complete consciousness returned only at the end of an hour. Much experimental work had still to be done before a surgeon could achieve easily, and with any degree of certainty, a steady and sustained period of unconsciousness, and, in fact, Morton's work still continues, for even today absolute safety is not assured.

While working on these technical problems Morton redoubled his efforts to publicize his discovery. He was quick to advertise his success, for he knew that his whole livelihood depended upon keeping ahead. Although he had discovered something of such vast importance, he was a small-town dentist and continued to act like one. In America devotion to material interests was an essential part of the nation's philosophy, for, in Walt Whitman's words, "the extreme business energy, and this almost maniacal appetite for wealth" was considered "part of amelioration and progress". Morton began collecting testimonials in the usual fashion. The one from Warren, dated October 17th, read: "I hereby certify that I have twice seen the administration of Dr Morton's application for the prevention of pain; that it had a decided effect in preventing the suffering of the patient during operations, and that no bad consequences followed."

Dr Hayward gave him a similar testimonial for the patient from whom he had removed a tumour, and Dr Heywood certified that both patients had undergone operations without suffering". Still none of the doctors knew what Morton's preparation actually contained, for the aromatics successfully disguised the smell of the ether.

Morton also had a testimonial circular issued which said that he had discovered a compound by inhaling which a person was thrown into a sound sleep and rendered insensible to pain, that he had administered it in his own practice to extract teeth, and for surgical operations at the Massachusetts General Hospital, and in every case with the most complete success. On Saturday, October 17th, the first newspaper story appeared in the Boston *Daily Journal*, under the headline "Successful Operation!" On October 21st the Boston *Medical and Surgical Journal* had an article saying, "Strange stories are circulating in the papers of a wonderful preparation in this city by administering which a patient is affected for long enough to undergo operation without pain."

But Morton's chief concern at all times was to save humanity pain. He wanted his new treatment to be used as soon as possible, and to ensure that there was nowhere in America, or indeed, in the world, where they had not heard of his great discovery and did not know in exact detail his method of administration. In his ideas on publicity he was also ahead of his time, for he promptly embarked on a grandiose scheme to launch his painless surgery, writing and issuing pamphlets advertising his new preparation, and getting famous doctors to attest to its efficacy in saving patients pain and allowing surgeons to go about their task unhindered. He worked hard too perfecting his apparatus and arranging for his inhaler to be reproduced in large quantities. He also set about establishing a regular supply of pure ether, and finally tackled the task of ensuring that his preparation would be administered correctly. He knew that the effects could be dangerous in unskilled and inexperienced hands, and he wanted to be certain that the best method and also the difficulties and dangers were known to all who wanted to try his new treatment. To this end he proposed to set up a clinic to study the subject and to publish an initial pamphlet explaining his method, and afterwards to issue further weekly bulletins giving the latest information. In this way he hoped to direct the development of the new pain-killer and to solve any problems which might arise during its use in different operations throughout the world.

The matter had now become much too big for Morton to handle personally, and he set to work to appoint agents to see that his new preparation was used only by properly trained people, to handle the patent, and to represent his interests throughout the world. Morton immediately thought of his old partner Wells, who had abandoned dentistry and was at that time organizing a "Scientific Panorama" exhibition. He wrote to him on October 19th:

FRIEND WELLS: DEAR SIR,
I write to inform you that I have discovered a preparation by inhaling which a person is thrown into a sound sleep. The time required to produce sleep is only a few moments, and the time in which persons remain asleep can be regulated at pleasure. While in this state the severest surgical or dental operations may be performed, the patient not experiencing the slightest pain.

I have perfected it, and am now sending out agents to dispose of the right to use it. I will dispose of the right to an individual to use it in his own practice alone, or for a town, county or state.

My object in writing to you is to know if you would not like to visit New York and other cities to dispose of rights upon shares. I have used the compound in more than one hundred and sixty cases in extracting teeth, and I have been invited to administer it to patients in the Massachusetts General Hospital and have succeeded in every case.

The Professors Warren and Hayward have given me certificates to this effect. I have administered it in the hospital in the presence of students and physicians—the room for operating being as full as possible. For further particulars, I refer you to extracts from the daily journals of this city, which I forward to you.[4]

Although it was something that Wells had himself attempted so unsuccessfully, he did not begrudge Morton his success, and there was no rancour in his reply:

DOCTOR MORTON: DEAR SIR,
Your letter dated yesterday is just received, and I hasten to answer it, for I fear you will adopt a method of disposing of your rights which will defeat your object. Before you make any arrangements whatever, I wish to see you. I think I will be in Boston the first of next week, probably on Monday night. If the operation of administering the gas is not attended with too much trouble, and will produce the effect you state, it will, undoubtedly, be a fortune to you, provided it is rightly managed.
Yours in haste,
H. WELLS[5]

Morton's was an ambitious scheme, designed to control the use of his preparation throughout the world, and certainly expensive to operate. He intended to cover these costs by selling licences to use his preparation and by a royalty on the price of all inhalers. He offered licences to doctors and dentists, the price depending upon the size of the localities in which they practised. In towns with a population of 5000 to 10,000 inhabitants he asked dentists fifty dollars for a five-year period. In cities of more than 100,000 inhabitants he asked 2000 dollars for a three-year period. Surgeons
80

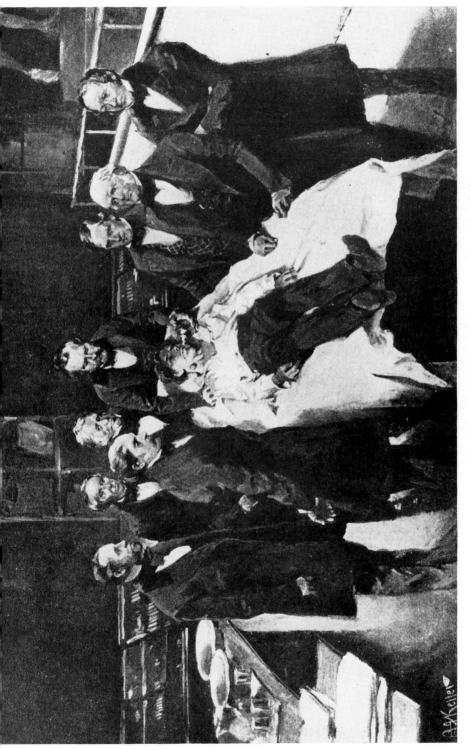

Painting commemorating the operation on Abbott on October 16th, 1846

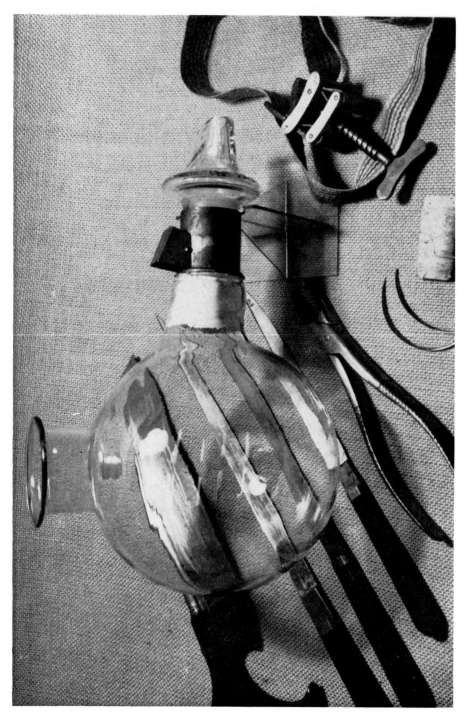

One of the first inhalers, and instruments used at that time were to pay 25 per cent of the fees they received for operations in which Morton or one of his trained men administered his preparation.

Morton was carried along on the tide of enthusiasm and initial success of his discovery, but knew that eventually it all depended upon getting a patent. He had already given notice on October 1st, the day after the extraction of Frost's tooth, but at that time R. H. Eddy, a local lawyer who acted as the Commissioner of Patents, was not certain whether it would be possible to grant one for a preparation consisting of only one substance and being used for such a purpose. Patents were granted under a Bill signed by George Washington in 1790 to protect the right of an inventor of "any useful art, manufacture, engine, machine or device, or any improvement thereon not before known or used", and Eddy had now been advised by Charles M. Keller, an illustrious Washington lawyer, that in his opinion Morton's discovery was as patentable as Watt's invention of the steam-engine. Daniel Webster, the famous lawyer and politican, endorsed this opinion, and when Morton went to see Eddy on October 21st he was delighted to hear from him that it was possible to take out a patent for his discovery.

Morton was relieved that his discovery would now be protected, for he had already made so many plans, and all depended upon the patent. As time went on he had become more and more worried that people would find out the contents of his preparation, for although it was still supposed to be a secret some of his friends had guessed from his experiments and from what he had told them that it contained some ether. Gould was already supposed to have blurted this out to Jackson.

Only two days after Eddy had told him that his discovery could be patented Morton was surprised to receive a visit from Jackson. It was the first time he had seen him since the 1st of October, when Jackson had refused to give him a certificate for his discovery. Jackson remarked that he had just looked in to see how he was getting on. He said that he had been informed by Eddy that a patent for the discovery was about to be taken out from which a great deal of money would be made, and as he had never before made any charge or received any recompense for the medical instruction he had rendered, he thought he must charge something—say, 500 dollars for it. Morton must have looked astonished, for Jackson remarked immediately that "he had been disappointed in his receipts for that year, and was obliged to look a little more carefully to his money matters in consequence of it". "As the patent will be exceedingly valuable to you, why," he added, "cannot a compensation be made from the receipts from that?"[6]

Morton could hardly believe his ears, for only three weeks before Jackson had flatly refused to give Morton a certificate for his preparation, or to allow his name to be connected with it. Now here he was demanding some of the proceeds. Jackson's first reaction had been to have nothing at all to do with it, for he believed, like the other authorities at that time, that if ether inhalation were to be prolonged, death would inevitably result. Now that Morton had shown pain could be eliminated with little danger to the patient, and after the leading surgeons had given him their support, Jackson's attitude had changed. When he heard from Eddy that a great deal of money was likely to be made out of the patent he had changed his tune. Apparently all he wanted now was to grab what he could of the profits.

Certainly Morton was surprised by his demand, and anyway regarded 500 dollars as an exorbitant fee for such simple advice, advice which any skilled chemist would have given him free. But Morton did not want to be bothered with any arguments with Jackson; he was very busy, and just wanted to be allowed to get on with his work. He had no money to give Jackson right away, but if the patent did succeed he did not mind giving his old tutor 10 per cent of the profits up to 500 dollars. He was grateful to Jackson for his help and advice in the past, and was happy to help him over what Jackson had told him was a lean period.

The next day Morton went to Eddy's. Jackson had asked Morton to meet him there to sign the papers to pay him his 500 dollars. Dana and Gould had come along to act as witnesses, but to everyone's surprise Jackson raised so many objections that the matter had to be postponed until the following day. What Morton did not know was that Eddy and Jackson had discussed the agreement together privately several times already. Richard Eddy was a local solicitor, and he and Jackson and their families were great friends. When the patent had first been issued Eddy had gone round to tell Jackson and to suggest that he take a part in the patent. At that time Jackson was afraid to be connected with the discovery for fear there might be a fatal accident and his good name prejudiced, but in any case, according to Eddy, he "thought the matter of little value". He told Eddy that Morton had already agreed to pay him 500 dollars and that he would be quite satisfied if he got that. (A lie actually, for Jackson did not ask Morton for money until the day after.)

On the evening of Friday, October 23rd, after he had seen Morton, Jackson and his wife and mother-in-law were visiting Eddy's father, Caleb. When Jackson grandly claimed the credit for suggesting the ether to Morton, Caleb then asked him the question which was to become famous:

"Did you know at such time, that, after a person had inhaled ether and was asleep, his flesh could be cut with a knife without his experiencing any pain?"

"No!" Jackson retorted, "nor Morton either; he is a reckless man for using it as he has; the chance is he will kill somebody yet."[7]

Richard Eddy himself had been to the theatre that night to see the Keans in *The Wife's Secret* and returned to find the Jackson family in his father's drawing-room. He told Jackson that the patent looked like earning a lot of money and again urged him to ask for a share of Morton's patent. But Jackson was still worried. Although Morton had proved it safe, he told Eddy he dare not be associated with the patent because the laws of Massachusetts Medical Society strictly forbade doctors to deal "in secret remedies". Eddy stressed that as part-owner of the patent he would stand to get a share of the cash, but if he kept out he would lose as he had done with Morse and his electric telegraph. (Morse's invention was a very sore point with Jackson, for he still clung to his story that he was the rightful discoverer.) Mrs Jackson also backed Eddy in his attempt to persuade her husband to ask for a share in the patent, but in spite of their efforts Jackson still hesitated. It seemed to be a case of sour grapes, for although he was plainly envious of Morton's great success, he thought he was forbidden by his profession to take part, and had gone round saying that Morton was nothing but a little commercially minded dentist and that he might do what he pleased with his patent for all he cared.

But the thought that Morton might make a lot of money obviously rankled in his mind, and by the following day, October 24th, when he went to see Eddy to sign the legal documents, Jackson had already had second thoughts. He arrived early to discuss the matter further before the others came, and Eddy again gave his opinion that Morton would stand to make a great deal of money from the sale of his licences. He pointed out, too, that as Jackson was an old friend of his he would very much like to see him getting some part of the bonanza. Jackson's greedy instincts were now thoroughly aroused. He was looking desperately for some way to get round the rules of the Medical Society, and decided to play for more time to consider the matter again. When the others arrived, much to Morton's surprise, Jackson made so many objections to the form of agreement that they had to leave the signing of the documents until the following day.

After the meeting Jackson went over the patent again with Eddy. It was undoubtedly a difficult situation, but if the patent was going to produce the large sums of money that Eddy expected Jackson wanted to get hold of a share of it. But he was bound firmly by the ethics of the medical profession, and as a physician of high standing he was forbidden to keep secret any remedy he discovered. He dared not risk being expelled by the Medical Society. Would it not be better, he asked, to stick to a cash settlement and to leave the patent to Morton and let him cope with all the responsibilities it would entail and the difficulties of enforcement?

Still Jackson found the vast profits tempting. He asked Eddy if he would go round and discuss the matter with Gould, who was a doctor and a friend of Jackson's. There Gould showed Eddy a copy of the by-laws of the Medical Society, and they went through them together. Gould thought Jackson's fears were groundless, for the rules of the Society were extremely flexible. Jackson was not a practising physician, and there would therefore be no difficulty about taking a share in the patent. Eddy himself had also already put forward a strictly legal view that once the patent was granted it could no longer be said to be secret, for the very derivation of the word patent stemmed from the Latin *patere*, to lie open. Jackson, of course, was only too anxious to find some way round the difficulty, and when he heard their views he is reported to have said, "Well, if Dr Gould thinks so, that settles the matter. I have no objection to signing." Straight away he instructed Eddy to inform Morton that for his part in the discovery he insisted upon having 10 per cent of all patent revenues, even beyond the 500 dollars.

Morton was staggered when Eddy told him of Jackson's demand, and even more amazed when Eddy also advised him to include Jackson in the patent. Morton assured him that although Jackson had given him some technical advice, he was certainly not in any way connected with his discovery. He had been using ether in his experiments long before he saw Jackson, and he strongly repudiated Jackson's assertion that he was now entitled to 10 per cent of his patent. He had consulted Dr Jackson only as an expert chemist, and he was most indignant at Jackson's claim.

Eddy was puzzled at the way the affair was developing. Jackson was a great friend of his and a famous and highly respected scientist. Morton, on the other hand, was a little-known dentist with no qualifications or education, and Eddy naturally was more inclined to believe Jackson. "Dr Jackson and I, during this period, were on very strong friendly terms. I entertained for him the purest feelings of amity, and was ever ready to do him, or the members of his family, any favour in my power. I have reason to believe, I had with him the position of a confidential and very intimate friend."[8] This readiness to do his old and respected friend any favour influenced him greatly in his efforts to persuade Morton to give Jackson his 10 per cent. "In rendering such advice," said Eddy, "I was fully impressed with the belief from the statement of Dr Jackson that he had suggested to Dr Morton the propriety of experimenting with ether; and that Dr Morton, without the presence or further assistance of Dr Jackson, had practically demonstrated the effect of ether to annul pain. Upon this I reasoned that, had Dr Morton kept the discovery secret, neither Dr Jackson nor the world would have known of the result; or, in other words, had not Dr Morton performed the experiment he did, the discovery could not have taken place. . . . It seemed to me a clear case of joint discovery." Eddy's excuse later for this fatal error of judgement was that he could never get a chance to talk to Morton, for "whenever he went to his surgery it was always thronged with people" waiting for Morton's attention.

Morton was incensed. He had already agreed to pay Jackson the 500 dollars, and that was more than enough. Eddy suggested that Morton would do well to avoid a disagreement with Jackson, even if strictly speak-

84

ing he had no legal right to the 10 per cent, and argued circumspectly that if Morton gave him (Eddy) 25 per cent and Jackson 10 per cent of all the revenues even beyond the 500 dollars they would be able to conduct the business of the patent and save Morton the bother of it. Eddy was obviously trying to get the best deal for his old friend Jackson, and for himself too, and was concerned more to see that they made as much money as possible out of the patent than he was about Morton's real interests.

Still Morton insisted that Jackson had no right to a percentage of his patent. He was happy to give Eddy his 25 per cent as a recompense for his services, but he refused absolutely to give Jackson another cent beyond the 500 dollars already agreed. Eddy continued to press Jackson's case, arguing that he had often seen applications for patents dismissed because of personal disputes between the applicants. He advised Morton to settle the question amicably, for otherwise Jackson might try to stop the patent being granted, pressing Morton "lest the aid he had given me might be made a handle of by persons impeaching the patent, to invalidate my claim as discoverer."[9] He argued too that "the patent would have the benefit of Dr Jackson's name and skill", and thus the importance of Morton's discovery was likely to be recognized far sooner. Jackson would also prove a good witness if ever a case were to be brought against him, and his chemical knowledge would be available, for he would "have a motive to give his attention to the preparation and the apparatus"[10] and to help promote and develop the discovery.

Eddy's arguments at last began to tell on Morton. After all, he told himself, Eddy was a well-educated man, respected in the community, and a lawyer with great experience of patent cases. On the other hand, he himself was just a young, uneducated dentist who had been forced to make his own way in the world. With no knowledge or experience of legal affairs and at a disadvantage among such educated men as Jackson and Eddy, he said, "I felt the need of all the aid I could get and was conscious of a want of thorough scientific education myself."[11]

When Gould, a clever doctor and a friend of his, also advised him to give Jackson what he asked Morton decided to stifle his indignation at the injustice of it and to let Jackson have his paltry 10 per cent. He had no wish to quarrel with him. He was not an ungenerous man. All he wanted was to be left to get on with his plans for the whole world to benefit from his discovery of painless surgery.

But the die was cast and the damage done, and the effects of this simple action were to be disastrous.

NOTES TO CHAPTER VIII

1. *McClure's Magazine*, September 1896.
2. *The Lancet*, I, 1847.
3. *Ibid.*
4. Nathan Rice, *Trials of a Public Benefactor*.
5. *Ibid.*
6. *Ibid.*
7. *Littell's Living Age*, 1848.
8. Nathan Rice, *op. cit.*
9. *Ibid.*
10. *Ibid.*
11. *Ibid.*

CHAPTER

IX

WHEN Wells came to Boston Morton demonstrated his preparation to him, but Wells "expressed himself alarmed, said I should kill someone yet and break myself up in business". They discussed the possibilities of his discovery, but Wells thought that Morton would be unable to secure a patent, and with his usual 'get-rich-quick' mentality he advised Morton to "make as much money as possible by selling as many licences as possible while the application is pending and the excitement is high". Morton did his best to persuade Wells to become one of his agents, but Wells thought that the future prospects of the patent were not good and declined his offer. Eddy also pressed Wells, but he was off to make his fortune in Paris and planned to leave as soon as possible.

But not everyone was as sceptical as Wells, and Morton's schemes were going ahead well. On October 29th Eddy set in motion plans to obtain patent rights abroad, and Morton asked Warren to supply him with a list of hospitals and charitable trusts so that he could grant them licences free. So far the contents of his preparation were not publicly known, for it was believed to be composed of several different substances. Warren now wanted to use the new treatment for all operations at the hospital, but Chamberlain told everyone that he could not supply inhalers without Morton's authorization. The inhaler had been invented by him and a patent applied for, and if the doctors wanted to buy them they must get Morton's permission first. Warren himself was quite prepared to pay Morton for the use of his inhaler, for it was of the utmost value to his patients, and he did not see any reason why the inventor should not gain from his discovery.

But if Warren saw no reason to object the Massachusetts Medical Society certainly did. The moment it was known that Morton had invented a marvellous pain-killer and was going to take out a patent for it he was heavily criticized. Medical ethics forbid the concealment of new discoveries and demand that they be given free to the world. Although Morton was not a member of the medical profession and not bound at all by any of their conventions, the members of the Society made no secret of the fact that even if they had no control over him, they could certainly stop any of the doctors or surgeons from using his discovery. They grumbled that something must be done at once to put an end to the scandal, for they were not going to allow Professor Warren to become a tool of this avaricious little dentist. Jealous of the young man's great success, they resented having to pay, while their colleagues at the hospital used Morton's discovery free. Although they admitted that Morton was quite at liberty to use a patented preparation in dentistry, now he was meddling in medical matters, they insisted that he must abide by their rules.

The matter came to a head early in November. At a special meeting of the Society they agreed that if Morton insisted on using the invention for private profit, then the Massachusetts medical practitioners must refuse to allow it to be used in their operations. The resolution was carried unanimously, and the staff of the Massachusetts General Hospital were officially notified of the decision. The decision came as a blow to Warren, for he had a special case in mind for the next painless-surgery operation—a woman of twenty-one, Alice Mohan, who had entered hospital on March 7th, 1845, with a diseased knee-joint, and now after all this time was to have her leg amputated. It was a far more formidable and painful operation than those for which Morton's preparation had previously been used, and if the method proved successful in this major operation, then the world could no longer doubt the magnitude of Morton's discovery.

Warren felt it was a pity that just at this crucial moment there should have been an argument about the patent. He himself was motivated by the noblest professional ideals, and as one of the founders of the hospital had played a major part in securing a medical profession based on the highest principles and practice. Nevertheless he felt it foolish to allow strict medical etiquette to stand in the way of one of the greatest discoveries ever made, and questioned the wisdom of the Society in raising the matter just then. Were surgeons to be forced to continue their terrible tortures in spite of what had happened at the momentous operation on October 16th? Through no fault of her own was poor Alice Mohan to be made to suffer the agonizing pain just because of a lot of small Boston doctors? At the same time Warren knew that if he chose to disregard the unanimous decision of the Medical Society he himself would be forbidden to go on practising, and therefore wrote to Morton informing him that the surgeons of the hospital thought it their duty to decline the use of the preparation until told what it contained. In an effort to meet the requirements of the Medical Society Morton replied to Warren on November 5th, 1846:

88

DEAR SIR,

As it may sometimes be desirable that surgical operations should be performed at the Massachusetts General Hospital under the influence of the preparation employed by me for producing temporary insensibility to pain, will you allow me, through you, to offer to the hospital the free use of it for all the hospital operations? I should be pleased to give the surgeons of the hospital any information, in addition to what they now possess, which they may think desirable in order to employ it with confidence. I will also instruct such persons as they may select, connected with the hospital, in the mode of employing it. This information, I must request, should be regarded as confidential, as I wish for ample time to make such modifications as experience may suggest in its exhibition. It is also my intention to have persons suitably instructed, who will go wherever desired, for a reasonable compensation, and administer it for private operations, thus enabling any surgeon to employ it in his private practice whenever he may have occasion. I think you will agree with me that this will be wiser until its merits are fuller established, than to put it into the hands of everybody, thereby bringing discredit upon the preparation by its injudicious employment. Should you wish me to administer at any of the operations tomorrow, I shall do so with pleasure; and should the above proposition be deemed worthy of being entertained, I shall be ready to make the arrangement as soon as informed of your wishes.

W. T. G. MORTON[1]

It was a magnanimous gesture, but still did not actually specify the contents of the preparation. Warren hoped that Morton's letter would meet the Society's point and wrote back:

DEAR SIR,

I beg to acknowledge the reception of your polite letter. I shall lose no time in laying it before the surgeons of the hospital.[2]

The date of the operation on Alice Mohan was now fixed for November 7th, 1846. It was announced in Boston newspapers, and the doctors of the city and from places quite far afield waited in great excitement. Dr G. M. Angell of Atlanta, who was on a visit to Boston at the time, described what happened:

On the morning of the day set for the operation, I went as usual to the hospital, but much earlier, as I anticipated from the great reputation of Dr Warren and the importance attached to the experiment that there would be a large attendance at the clinic. When I arrived, a very large crowd had already assembled in front of the hospital, reaching out to the sidewalk and street, but the door was kept closed until the usual hour of opening arrived. I passed in by a private door with a student: we went directly to the operating-room and chose our seats close to the railing and directly opposite to the operating theatre and impatiently awaited events. When the hour arrived and the doors were opened, the

89

great hall was filled to overflowing with the rushing host, which filled the seats and aisles to their utmost capacity.

But Dr Angell and the rest of the assembled crowd were forced to wait a long time, for behind the scenes a fierce battle was raging. Morton had not been asked to administer his preparation, and on the morning of the operation was still waiting at his house for word from the doctors. Bigelow came to call for him in his chaise to ask him to go with him to the hospital with his inhaler, for he wanted Morton on hand in case the doctors had a last-minute change of heart and decided to let him administer his preparation after all. When they got to the hospital Bigelow left Morton in the small room next to the dispensary and went to join the members of the Massachusetts Medical Society already assembled in the anteroom arguing furiously.

The meeting had begun with the members of the Society not on the staff of the hospital asking Dr Warren the simple question as to whether he was acquainted with the composition of the remedy with the aid of which he intended to perform this operation. Warren had replied that he was not, but, other than establishing that it was free from risk, he saw no reason for asking. In that case, replied the Vice-President of the Society, they would have to forbid Warren to use it, for they insisted that the fact that Morton had agreed to supply his preparation and apparatus free to hospitals still did not meet the requirements of their faculty. Medical men had the right, and indeed, the duty, to know the composition of all the medicines they used, for secret remedies were the device of quacks and responsible medical practitioners must have nothing to do with them. What they said was absolutely right, but patent medicines continue to thrive and doctors to prescribe them. Laudable though their pronouncements sounded, they also concealed less high-minded motives like fear and jealousy, and resentment at having to pay Morton for the use of his preparation. They knew that they had no power over him, but insisted that as a member of the Society Dr Warren dare not ignore their decision. If Morton did not reveal the contents of his preparation, then the operation must proceed without the benefit of his discovery. If he did not submit to their request, then Alice Mohan and all the other patients must suffer the terrors of the knife just as they had done before.

While Warren and Bigelow and the doctors argued Morton sat alone waiting anxiously. It seemed so unjust that after all his years of hard work, the great expense, and the agony and worry of discovering and developing his preparation, he was now to be allowed no recompense. Certainly he wanted the whole world to benefit from his great discovery, but he believed, too, that it was essential to retain the strictest control. If he declared the contents openly, how could he stop people misusing his preparation? It could be mishandled and the idea completely discredited.

90

It could prove dangerous and patients be killed. He had worked so hard for this moment, and it saddened him to think that his marvellous discovery might now be wrested from him. When he had begun his experiments he had been a successful dentist with a good income and a solid practice. To develop his discovery he had neglected his work and alienated his patients. If they took his patent from him he would be forced to return to being a dentist, but in a precarious financial and physical state and much worse off than before he had begun his experiments.

As he mused Bigelow returned to tell him that the surgeons had decided not to use his preparation, their objection being that the professional rule regarding the use of secret remedies forbade them to have anything to do with it. He said, "by way of encouragement, that he should urge it, by every means in his power, but that no disappointment must be felt in case of failure", and returned again to the doctors. Left alone, Morton continued to indulge in further bitter reflections on those strict rules of etiquette which could not be made to yield to the claims of suffering humanity. If he chose to go on with his patent and to keep his discovery solely for use in dental practices he could become a rich man. But if he gave it to the world he would become just a penniless dentist.

Inside the operating theatre the crowd still sat waiting impatiently. An hour had passed. The patient had not been brought in. The door to the anteroom remained firmly shut. The distinguished gathering had become impatient at the delay, and some began to drum their feet on the floor and to curse the waste of their time on such a worthless project.

In another room the patient, Alice Mohan, lay on a couch waiting for the operation to begin. All this time she had been lying desperately worrying, in frightened anticipation of the ghastly event to come. It seemed unlikely that she would have the benefit of Morton's discovery, and the doctors had already given her a dose of one hundred drops of laudanum. But it could do little to assuage the terrible torture she must inevitably suffer when Warren began to operate, torture to which the honourable members of the Medical Society had so readily condemned her.

Morton was almost frantic at the thought of her unnecessary agony. Much as he wanted to keep his preparation secret, how could he possibly allow her to suffer such agonizing pain when it was within his power to prevent it? The selfish, unfeeling members of the Medical Society might condemn her to her sufferings—he could not stop them, but he could not himself refuse to take the vital step to save her. When Bigelow returned he explained to Morton what had happened and how he had told the doctors that he thought Morton's letter would meet their objections. Dr Warren had read out the statement offering any further information that they thought desirable, and the announcement seemed to have been the turning-point. Bigelow had come back now to ask Morton if he would comply. Morton knew already what his answer must be. While he had been waiting there all that time he had made up his mind, and he followed Bigelow back up the stairs to the anteroom. Standing there before that crowd of doctors, all anxious to know his discovery and doubtless hoping to make some profit out of it for themselves—men to whom his own great struggles were of no consequence—he announced quietly and dramatically that the agent he had employed was ether. He stood there before them and humbly asked to be allowed to continue his experiments at the hospital. The doctors gave their consent. The operation could begin.

Inside the operating theatre annoyance and impatience gave way to excitement as the door opened and Alice Mohan was wheeled in, followed by the doctors. Dr George Hayward announced to the crowded room: "With the approval of the medical faculty of Boston, the patient, Alice Mohan, will inhale a vapour competent to allay the pain of the operation. The fluid whose vapour will be used is sulphuric ether."

Dr Warren explained the patient's medical history which now necessitated the removal of her leg. Morton stepped forward and put the inhaler to the patient's mouth. She coughed somewhat at first and complained she could not inhale because of the pungency of the ether, but soon fell into a gentle sleep. Bigelow checked her pulse, while Hayward drew a pin from his lapel. He stuck it into her arm. There was no reaction. He picked up the knife and went rapidly to work. Just as he was finishing Alice Mohan groaned, turning her head from side to side. Hayward bent down and took hold of her sleeve, calling her name. She looked up at him, still dazed.

"I guess you've been asleep, Alice," he said.

"I think I have, sir," she replied.

"Well, we brought you here for an amputation; are you ready?"

"Yes, sir," she said, "I am ready."

He reached out, picked up the bloody dismembered limb, showed it to her, and said gently, "It is all done."

The scene which followed was one of pandemonium. Men were beside themselves with joy, clapping their hands, stamping, and shouting. So ended the first painless major amputation. Morton described it in his usual modest fashion: "I administered the ether with perfect success. This was the first case of amputation." All went well, and Alice Mohan was discharged from the hospital on December 22nd, 1846. Amid the excitement the rancour was forgotten, but, as Bigelow observed, if anything had gone wrong and the patient had died it was Morton who would have been indicted for manslaughter, not the members of the Medical Society, who had sat there so comfortably and self-righteously in their seats.

Now there could be no doubt that Morton's discovery had achieved its purpose. The effectiveness was even more amply demonstrated in the operations which followed. In one of them Morton was called upon to administer the ether to an old man paralysed through spinal disease. The

92

treatment then to prevent it spreading was to cauterize each side of the vertebral column. How it could have been carried out before Morton's discovery is beyond belief, for even under ether a description makes the blood run cold. Morton first gave his preparation, then the surgeon took up the white-hot irons and "passed them over the tender white skin. There was a hiss; the flesh, blackened by the intensity, shrank crisply away, without a groan or a moan from the patient."[3]

Since the contents of his preparation had now been disclosed and the patent secured, a spate of articles appeared. Bigelow had given a brief statement to the American Academy of Arts and Sciences on November 3rd, 1846. Morton now consented to a more detailed account of his re-markable preparation, and on November 9th Bigelow read a long paper to the Boston Society of Medical Improvement. A report was printed in the Boston *Daily Advertiser* the next day. Warren added his comments:

> A new era has opened to the operating surgeon. His visitations on the most delicate parts are performed, not only without the agonizing screams he has been accustomed to hear, but sometimes with a state of perfect insensibility, and occasionally even with an expression of pleasure on the part of the patient. That is the most amazing miracle of all. Who could have imagined that drawing a knife over the delicate skin of the face might produce a sensation of unmixed delight? That the turning and twisting of instruments in the most sensitive parts might be accompanied by a delightful dream? If Ambroise Paré and Louis, and Dessault and Cheselden, Cooper and Hunter could see what our eyes daily witness, how would they long to come among us and perform their exploits once more. It is the most valuable discovery ever made, because it frees suffering humanity from pain. Unrestrained and free as God's own sunshine, it has gone forth to cheer and gladden the earth; it will awaken the gratitude of the present and of all coming generations. The student who from distant lands or in distant ages may visit this spot will view it with increased interest, as he remembers that here was first demonstrated one of the most glorious truths of science.[4]

No one at the time could have doubted Professor Warren's eulogy of Morton. All of Boston felt proud that the operation had taken place in their city, and Morton became its favourite son. Day after day the Press was full of articles glorifying the discovery, and scientists vied with one another to describe it in glowing terms. Oliver Wendell Holmes, himself a physician, and a poet and novelist, in one of his popular lectures claimed: "Nature herself is working out the primal curse which doomed the tenderest of her creatures to the sharpest of her trials, but the fierce ex-tremity of suffering has been steeped in the waters of forgetfulness, and the deepest furrow in the knotted brow of agony has been smoothed for ever."[5]

It was not only in Boston that there was acclamation, for, as Bigelow said after watching the first painless amputation, it was a shot that would soon echo around the world. Within a few days a New York journal wrote: "God bless the inventor of this last gift to man. It is the most glorious, nay, the most God-like discovery of this or any other age."[6] The news took longer to travel by steamship to Europe, but word reached England about three weeks later. Dr Jacob Bigelow, Henry's father and the renowned Boston physician, had written on November 28th to Dr Francis Boott, an American friend of his living in London, to tell him the startling news of Morton's great discovery, "which promises to be one of the most important discoveries of the present age. . . . The inventor is Dr Morton, a dentist of this city." He enclosed a copy of the article written by his son describing the operations in detail and the letter was read out to a meeting of some of Boott's colleagues. Soon it was all round London. On Saturday, December 19th, a London dentist, James Robinson, extracted a tooth painlessly for Boott's niece.

Two days later, on Monday, December 21st, 1846, the famous surgeon Robert Liston was to carry out the first surgical operation to be performed in England under ether. Liston was acknowledged to be easily "the quickest man with the knife in England", for before Morton made his wonderful discovery speed was the measure of a surgeon's skill, and if he took too long the patient died from shock and pain. Six feet two inches tall, Liston was a massive, muscular giant of a man, said to unite the strength of a bear with the adroitness of a juggler, and stories of his exploits are legendary today. He loved his job and operated with great zest, applying his special long knife and giant saw with considerable relish. He disliked the smaller jobs of surgery, and one day when he was making a fuss about an eye operation being 'niggling' a patient at the other end of the ward asked why he was complaining so much. "Oh," said the head nurse, "Mr Liston likes something to carve at!"[7]

He must have looked a fearsome sight during operations, with his scalpel held between his teeth so that he had both hands free to tie off the blood-vessels. Once he had a patient who was so terrified that he ran away before he could be operated upon. Liston gave orders that next time he was not to be told the time of the operation. Still the man somehow got wind of it and ran and locked himself up in a lavatory. When Liston heard what had happened he sent for his long operating knife. Slipping back the bolt on the lavatory door, he flung it open to reveal the poor man, sitting there petrified with fear. Liston just picked him up by the seat of his breeches, ran him to the nearest table, strapped him down, and cut for the stone all in the short space of two minutes. Famous though he was for the lightning speed of his operations, he was supposed once to have been too quick in amputating a leg at the thigh, for he took off one of the man's testicles and two of his assistant's fingers at the same time!

This then was the great Liston, about to operate with ether for the first

94

time in England. It was a bitterly cold December, but the crowds lining the benches of the theatre at University College Hospital were more excited than cold, for word had gone round early that morning that Mr Liston intended to try something new. The students looked down on an operating theatre vastly different from today's, for most were furnished with just a small handbowl for the surgeon to wash off the blood spattered on him, an instrument cupboard, and in the centre the stark wooden operating table and chair, with a bench for visitors. At the foot of the operating table stood the usual box of sawdust ready for the surgeon to kick into place to catch the blood.

Presently the door opened, and William Squire, the apothecary's nephew, came in and started to set up the apparatus. Based on a description of Morton's inhaler, it was a Nooth's apparatus, the upper glass cylinder of which was packed with sponge, and attached to the lower a flexible tube with ordinary bronchial mouthpiece. Squire poured sulphuric

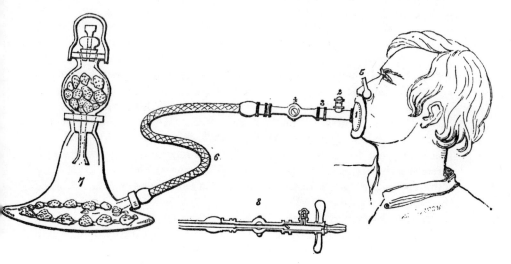

THE APPARATUS FOR RENDERING SURGICAL OPERATIONS PAINLESS.

THE NEW MEANS FOR RENDERING SURGICAL OPERATIONS PAINLESS.

LAST week, the first experiment was made in this country of employing the inhalation of the vapour of sulphur ether as a means of rendering surgical operations .

The first demonstration of the anaesthetic properties of ether in England following Morton's demonstration in America.
Illustrated London News, 1847.

95

ether on the sponge and asked for a volunteer to try it out, but no one would come forward. He looked round the room, and his eye lit on Sheldrake, a big, muscular attendant who was waiting at the door for Liston to arrive. He ordered the man to come forward, and reluctantly he came and lay down. He sucked at the inhaler while Squire held his nose but once again ether proved unpredictable, and after only one or two minutes' inhaling he suddenly became violent and leapt off the table, completely intoxicated. Pushing Squire roughly aside, Sheldrake clambered over the railings and plunged into the mass of students. The crowd separated right and left as he came at them, and for a while Sheldrake rushed on, almost to the door. There, as he paused a second to catch his breath, the students closed in and held him firmly until he had quietened down. Sheepishly he shuffled off down the stairs, swearing never to get caught again.

At a quarter past two Liston strode into the theatre, an enormous giant of a man, with a fierce and commanding presence, worshipped by his staff and students. With him was his assistant, William Cadge. They knew nothing of germs. Many of the students had come straight from the dissecting-room. Nobody thought about washing his hands before an operation, nobody took off his coat. Occasionally the surgeon would turn up his cuffs, but rarely the assistants. Liston wore an old, stained frockcoat, splattered and encrusted with the blood of countless patients who had lain before on that same operating table. He now took up from its case his long, narrow amputating knife. Specially made to his own design, the handle bore a number of notches—each like an Indian counting scalps, celebrating an operation at which the knife had previously been used. The house surgeon, Ransome, put out the saw, forceps, and the other simple instruments, pulled a few threads of waxed hemp ligature through his buttonhole, and stood ready to assist. Liston turned to the crowded theatre and announced, "We are going to try a Yankee dodge today, gentlemen, for making men insensible."[8]

The patient was brought in, a butler, Frederick Churchill, who had fallen and damaged his leg badly. The wound had suppurated and had been opened up again, and not surprisingly, after being exposed to these filthy hospital conditions, it had now gone putrescent and was to be amputated. He lay there on the table, pale and emaciated, wasted by the fever. A handkerchief was put over his face and the mouthpiece of the inhaler put underneath, but even so he cried out with fright as it was thrust into his mouth. Soon he began to relax.

Liston stood there watching him, quietly testing the blade of his knife with his thumb. Dressers stood by to hold down the patient, but this time their services were not necessary. Eventually Squire looked over to Liston and said, "I think he'll do, sir."

"Take the artery, Cadge," said Liston. Ransome held the limb. "Now, gentlemen, time me!" said Liston.

96

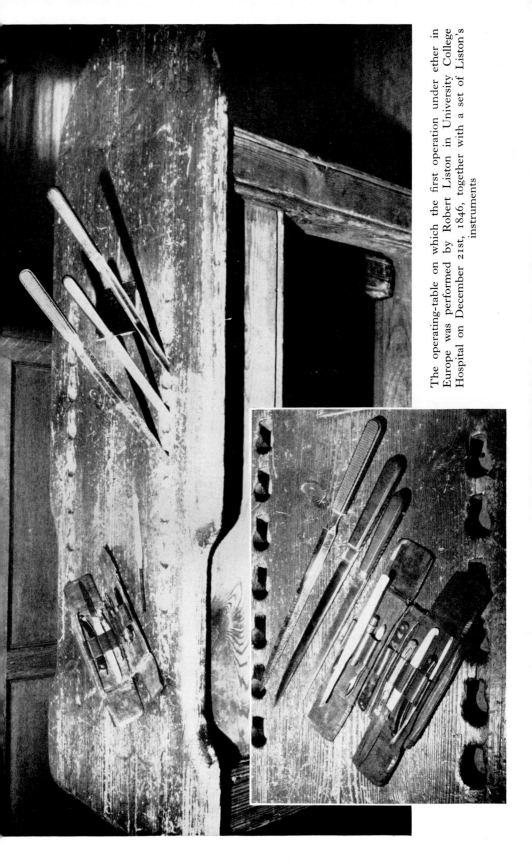

The operating-table on which the first operation under ether in Europe was performed by Robert Liston in University College Hospital on December 21st, 1846, together with a set of Liston's instruments

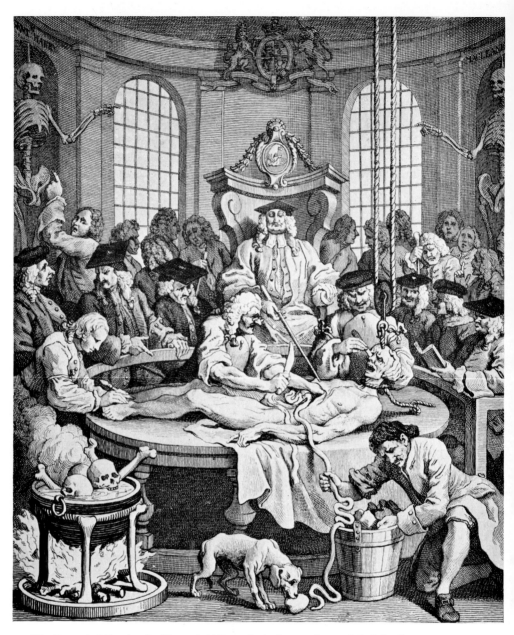

The Reward of Cruelty, by Hogarth (After criminals were hanged their bodies were used for dissection.)

This was one of his favourite gambits with his students, for he prided himself on his reputation. Scores of watches all over the theatre were soon pulled out and opened. His huge left hand grasped the thigh, a thrust of his long straight knife, a few quick flashes, half a dozen strokes of the saw, and Ransome tossed the leg into the sawdust.

"Twenty-eight seconds," said William Squire.

"Twenty-seven," said one of the students.

Liston's dresser beamed up at his master, "Twenty-five, sir!" he said.[9]

The handkerchief was removed from the man's face, and everyone stared in utter disbelief at the apparently gently sleeping patient. He began to recover. "Take me away, I can't have it off," he said, "I must die as I am."[10] They showed him the bloody stump, and he fell back sobbing on the pillow. Everyone present was greatly moved as the porters carried the man back to the ward, only five minutes or so after he had left it. Liston stood watching him go, the great Liston himself, almost overcome with fear and elation. Turning to the audience and stammering with his intense excitement, he exclaimed, "This Yankee dodge, gentlemen, beats mesmerism hollow!"[11]

In fact, only partial unconsciousness had actually been achieved, for the patient was reported to have answered questions on the operating table, and again it showed just how afraid the doctors were of giving too large a dose. For them deep and complete unconsciousness was the certain prelude to death, and it was this enormous barrier which had defied doctors and scientists for centuries, until Morton with great courage and inspiration had surmounted it to venture into unknown territory.

Liston was cock-a-hoop at his great success, and that night gave a dinner-party at his house at 5 Clifford Street, Old Bond Street, to celebrate the event. There he again demonstrated the effects of ether on his poor assistant, Cadge, for the benefit of his guests. The news of Liston's operation soon spread round London, and the *People's London Journal* wrote on January 9th, 1847:

> Hail, happy hour! that brings the glad tidings of another glorious victory. Oh, what a delight for every feeling heart to find the new year ushered in with the announcement of this noble discovery of the power to still the sense of pain and veil the eye and memory from all the horrors of an operation. . . . WE HAVE CONQUERED PAIN. That is, indeed, a glorious victory . . . the victory of knowledge over ignorance, of good over evil. . . . Benevolence has its triumph. It is a victory not for today, nor for our own time, but for another age, and all time; not for one nation, but for all nations, from generation to generation, as long as the world shall last.

The Lancet said, a little condescendingly, "that its discoverer should be an American is a high honour to our transatlantic brethren". In the English medical journals Morton was repeatedly compared with the celebrated

Jenner, and, indeed, there were striking similarities. Both were relatively uneducated men, and both had made two of the greatest contributions to medical science. Jenner had come to be regarded as almost a saint, and to be compared to him was indeed high praise.

Paris then was the great centre of medical learning and surgery, and might have been expected to be the least ready to accept new ways, for only a short time before one of the greatest surgeons of the nineteenth century, Louis Velpeau, had declared that pain and surgery were inseparable. Morton had sent off one of his inhalers to Willie Fisher, an American friend of his who lived in Paris, and also copies of the testimonials from Warren and Bigelow. Fisher was a Bostonian who was proud that this wonderful discovery should have been made in his native city, and after he had tried it out himself he took the inhaler round to the St Louis Hospital and gave a demonstration there to its surgeons. He persuaded them to try it out, and also Velpeau himself. Various operations were performed under ether, and the success was overwhelming. It was enthusiastically acclaimed in Germany, and again in Vienna: "This is the most important and greatest discovery of our century." In Russia it was "the greatest blessing, a gift from heaven".

So the news spread. Soon Morton's great discovery became known throughout the civilized world, and afterwards was carried by missionaries even into the remotest parts. His story should have ended in triumph, but the tragedy was yet to come.

NOTES TO CHAPTER IX

1. Nathan Rice, *Trials of a Public Benefactor*.
2. *Ibid.*
3. *Ibid.*
4. *Ibid.*
5. *Ibid.*
6. *Ibid.*
7. F. W. Cock, "The First Operation under Ether in England", in *American Journal of Surgery*, 29 (Anaesthesia Supplement), 1915.
8. *Ibid.*
9. *Ibid.*
10. Dr W. Squire, *The Lancet*, II, December 2nd, 1888.
11. *American Journal of Surgery*, 29 (Anaesthesia Supplement), 1915.

CHAPTER

ALTHOUGH his preparation was now known to contain only ether, Morton still went ahead with his plans. On November 12th, 1846, he was officially informed that he had been granted Patent No. 4848 for a period of fourteen years, under the patent system which Lincoln said added the fuel of interest to the fire of genius. He now joined those distinguished names among the three million patents granted in the United States up to the present day: Whitney for his cotton gin, McCormick for his reaper, two inventions which together laid the foundations of the United States economy; Morse for his electric telegraph; Colt and Gatling for their famous guns; Edison for his electric lamp; Ford for "new and useful improvements in motor carriages". Some, like Gidden's invention of barbed wire, have literally gone right round the world, while others have been as unknown as Mark Twain's "improvement in adjustable and detachable straps for garments" or Abraham Lincoln's "device for buoying vessels over shoals". Morton also applied for patents abroad, and sent Edward Warren—no relation to the Boston surgeon—to Europe to act as his agent. He applied for rights in France and several other countries, and on December 21st, 1846, a patent was granted in London and held by J. A. Dorr on Morton's behalf. When *The Lancet* carried an account of Liston's first painless operation Dorr wrote a letter to the editor:

> SIR,
>   Having noticed, in several periodicals and newspapers, reports of two operations recently performed by Mr Liston at the University College Hospital . . . I take this earliest opportunity of giving notice, through the medium of your columns, to the medical profession, and to the public in general, that the process of producing insensibility to pain by the administration of the vapour of ether to the lungs, employed by Mr

Liston, is patented for England and the Colonies, and that no person can use that process, or any similar one, without infringing upon rights, legally secured to others. . . .

JAMES A. DORR

DUKE STREET,
ST JAMES'S
December 28, 1846[1]

Morton was not the only one to realize the value of his discovery, for he was immediately approached by other dentists who hoped to make a profit too. One was Nathan C. Keep, Vice-President of the American Dental Association, who previously had sold his professional secrets to Morton for 500 dollars. Keep was a shrewd member of the profession who had always been very aware of the commercial possibilities of new forms of treatment. When he began his career Morton had considered it worth while to buy Keep's professional secrets—the tricks of the trade. Now the position was reversed, and it was Morton who was selling the use of his preparation. On November 28th they inserted an advertisement in the Boston *Evening Traveller*: "The subscribers, having associated themselves in the business of dental surgery, would respectfully invite their friends to call on them at their rooms, No. 19 Tremont Row; they confidently believe that the increased facilities which their united experience will afford them of performing operations with elegance and dispatch, and the additional advantage of having them performed without pain, by the use of the fluid recently invented by Dr Morton, will not only meet the wishes of their former patients, but secure them additional patronage."

Under their agreement Keep was to exploit the discovery in dentistry, while Morton was free to devote himself to developing it for the much more important use in surgery. His plans seemed to be going well, and he had notices inserted in various newspapers that letters patent had been granted and that suitable people could buy licences. He invited physicians, surgeons, and dentists who wanted to see for themselves the effect of his new treatment to call at his rooms. He also cautioned people against infringement of his patent if they wished to avoid the "trouble and expense of prosecution and damage at law". He wanted to keep it from the unskilled or ignorant, and warned that no one should trust themselves to the hands of those who did not have his permission to administer his apparatus and preparation. The theory of the patent law was that instead of keeping the invention secret for his own gain, the inventor disclosed it so that the public might benefit from it, and also could use it freely after the patent had expired. It was a system without which, one of Mark Twain's characters observed, the country was "just a crab and cannot travel anyway but sideways and backways". But although Morton continued in public the impossible battle of defending his patent, privately he was still worried about the ethical considerations of his actions and whether it was right to

100

limit the use of a preparation which could save humanity suffering. He had set out to find a way of eliminating pain so that he could crown defective teeth, and, like any other enthusiastic young dentist, to build up as large and as profitable a practice as possible and to provide for his young wife and family. As a dentist he was bound by no vows or conventions, and it was perfectly permissible for him to patent his discovery. His business instincts were those of Puritan New England, where zealous men strove to worship God and do his will in their daily life, secure in the belief that God would bless them in their business activities too. The virtuous were those most blessed with material wealth, and, as Emerson observed, "In a former age men of might were men of will, now they are men of wealth." Jay Cooke, the future financier of the Civil War, wrote home from Philadelphia about 1840: "Through all the grades I see the same all-pervading, all-engrossing anxiety to grow rich. This is the only thing for which men live here." He promised himself: "I shall . . . go into business myself, and live in palaces and castles which kings might own."

With material prosperity such a test of virtue, it would have been surprising had Morton not seen in his patent his chance to make a fortune and not been determined to hold on to it. As far as he was concerned he had made the discovery and the patent was his property. He came from a profession where they kept their new techniques to themselves, and it was hardly to be expected, therefore, that a small-town dentist like himself would easily relinquish his right to the patent.

The doctors might condemn him self-righteously, motivated too by jealousy, but the pages of medical history are strewn with examples of cures withheld until a fee had been paid. In the seventeenth century the Chamberlen family guarded the secret of their midwifery forceps, and even when at last the medical faculty of Amsterdam bought a poor copy they continued to drive a hard bargain, so that once more the women of the country were held to ransom, but this time by their own doctors. In more modern times discoveries made by doctors have soon been taken up by chemical industries, and profits from their manufacture have gone to swell private pockets. Domagk's discovery leading to the sulphonamide drugs was soon ringed round with patents, and although Fleming tried to avoid it, his great discovery of penicillin was eventually patented, as are the rest of the new wonder drugs.

James Dorr, Morton's patent agent in London, discussed the issues in his letter to the editor of *The Lancet* of December 28th, 1846: "I am aware that doubts exist in the minds of some as to the liberality of rendering inventions or improvements, which tend to alleviate suffering, subjects of patents; but I cannot see why the individual who, by skill and industry, invents or discovers the means of diminishing, or, as in this instance, annihilating human suffering, is not full as much entitled to compensation as he who makes an improvement in the manufacture of woollen or other

101

fabrics. Indeed, he is entitled to greater compensation, and for a stronger reason—he had conferred upon mankind a greater benefit."

Morton was, of course, not out simply to make money. The farther he had gone with his discovery, the more he had realized the immense value of it to mankind. He wanted the world to benefit, but hoped at the same time to get compensation for the expenses he had incurred. He talked to Warren and Bigelow and the other doctors, who were themselves still apprehensive about using ether, and even more concerned at what would happen if it were freely available to everyone. Bigelow set out his views in the paper given before the Boston Society for Medical Improvement, and afterwards circulated in America and the rest of the world, "upon the actual position of this invention as regards the public". He went on:

> No one will deny that he who benefits the world should receive from it an equivalent. The only question is, of what nature shall the equivalent be? Shall it be voluntarily ceded by the world, or levied upon it? For various reasons, discoveries in high science have been usually rewarded indirectly by fame, honour, position, and occasionally, in other countries, by funds appropriated for the purpose. Discoveries in medical science, whose domain approaches so nearly that of philanthropy, have been generally ranked with them; and many will assent with reluctance to the propriety of restricting by letters patent the use of an agent capable of mitigating human suffering. There are various reasons, however, which apologise for the arrangement, which I understand to have been made with regard to the application of the new agent.
>
> 1st. It is capable of abuse, and can readily be applied to nefarious ends.
> 2nd. Its action is not yet thoroughly understood, and its use should be restricted to responsible persons.
> 3rd. One of its greatest fields is the mechanical art of dentistry, many of whose processes are by convention, secret, or protected by patent rights. It is especially with reference to this art, that the patent has been secured. We understand, already, that the proprietor has ceded its use to the Massachusetts General Hospital, and that his intentions are extremely liberal with regard to the medical profession generally; and that as soon as necessary arrangements can be made for publicity of the process, great facilities will be offered to those who are disposed to avail themselves of what now promises to be one of the most important discoveries of the age.[2]

The ethics of patents are still argued around the world, but Bigelow reported that the decision had not been reached by Morton "without mature consideration on his part, and after conferring with several upon whose judgement he relied". Morton was urged even more strongly to restrain the use of such a powerful agent now that his preparation was generally known to be only ether, for he was advised that only through his patent would he be able to restrict its use to skilled and properly trained operators. But at the same time he announced on November 26th that he hoped the Government would take over his patent and allow it to be used freely for the public good, and if the Government did so he offered to repay any licence fees.

Still the tide of success did not run entirely with Morton. The bastions of tradition do not capitulate so easily, and even when some startling discovery has been made and its value so conclusively demonstrated, older heads are still shaken in dismay. Innovators are rarely received with joy, and established authorities launch into condemnation of newer truths, for, as Maeterlinck pointed out, at every crossroads to the future there are a thousand self-appointed guardians of the past. Even in the medical world where new ideas save lives, changes are made only in the teeth of the most ruthless opposition from reigning experts. When Lister put forward his new theories about germs he was savagely attacked by Simpson, then a revered figure in the medical world, and it took seventeen years before Lister's antiseptic methods were adopted in London. It is no wonder that the *People's London Journal* said about Morton's discovery: "And then to find it acted upon almost on the instant by our first operators, is as gratifying as unexpected."

Only by the determination of discoverers like Morton is progress ever made at all, for along with the acclamation his discovery received, he also had to face a virulent campaign of condemnation. At first it was only his fellow-dentists. Maddened and angry that Morton had got in ahead of them and by his patent retained control of his discovery, they began to attack him furiously. Frightened at the thought of losing their patients, jealous dentists banded themselves together to form a Committee of Vigilance presided over by Dr Josiah Foster Flagg, a Boston dentist, to fight against the "sinister new discovery". Any incident which could possibly point to failure was seized upon and exaggerated; every example of supposed damage was noted. Eventually they produced a report which was printed in the *Boston Daily Advertiser* and gave details of young ladies who had suffering bleeding from the lungs, and melancholia, and others who had been delirious for days after receiving Morton's treatment. The parents of a small boy testified that their son had been so ill after having a tooth painlessly extracted by Morton that they had been forced to call a doctor, who pronounced the child to have been poisoned. The Committee issued dire warnings obviously aimed at Morton, cautioning the public against unqualified dentists. Finally, they issued a manifesto to condemn the new treatment.

Soon the dentists were joined by diehards in the medical profession, and even *The Lancet* referred to it dubiously in its first reports as "more striking to the general than to the scientific mind", and added guardedly, "*if* his discovery stands the test of time". Some doctors, annoyed that their

103

colleagues in Boston had got in ahead of them, joined the opposition out of petty spite. "All the medical magazines in the Union, except Boston," says Morton, "were arrayed against it." The *Medical Examiner* of Philadelphia condemned his discovery as "a swindle" and "quackery", and wrote: "We should not consider it entitled to the least notice but that we perceive by the Boston Medical and Surgical Journal . . . that prominent members of the profession in that city . . . have been caught in its meshes." It was hoped that the surgeons of Philadelphia would not be "seduced from the high professional path of duty, into the quagmire of quackery, by this Will-o'-the Wisp".[3]

Old habits die hard, even when they are obviously inferior, and a dentist from Baltimore wrote saying: "I protest against the whole business, because I verily believe the great discovery to be utterly useless. If we are to induce insensibility, I very much prefer whisky punch to ether, because it is more certain and more permanent in its effect."[4] New York medical journals regretted that their professional colleagues in Boston should have "intercourse with, and become the abettors of, quackery".[5] The New Orleans *Medical Journal* added its voice to the clamour: "Why, mesmerism, which is repudiated by the SAVANTS of Boston, has done a thousand times greater wonders and without any of the dangers here threatened. . . . That the leading surgeons of Boston could be captivated by such an invention as this excites our amazement."[6]

Even the great French physiologist Magendie spoke out against what he termed "this accursed novelty", and poured scorn on those who shrank from inflicting pain, condemning it as immoral and unworthy to try by artificial sleep to transform the patient's body to "an insensitive corpse" before beginning to operate. Against such powerful voices as these Morton had to fight a slow and tiresome battle. Hospitals continued to boast that they had not tried ether for operations and even as late as 1868 *The Medical Times* reported that in many towns in France patients still suffered surgery without any anaesthetic.

The dentists and doctors opposing Morton were quickly joined by the religious, who declared that pain was given by God Himself and that any attempt to avoid it was to oppose God's will. Soon clergymen were to be heard thundering against ether from the pulpit and declaring, as they did against chloroform later, that, "It is a decoy of Satan . . . but in the end, it will harden society and rob God of the deep earnest cries which arise in time of trouble for help."[7]

The religious in turn were joined by a whole army of naturalists, crackpots, freemasons, and others objecting on false scientific grounds. Mrs Morton said: "Abuse and ridicule were showered upon him by the public press, from the pulpit, and also by prominent medical journals, for presuming or daring to claim that he could prevent the pain of surgical operations. In those days I feared to look into a newspaper, for what wife does

104

not feel more keenly unjust aspersions on her husband than he for himself? Then, too, the world's way—jealousy, malice, and envy—was new to me."[8]

Hundreds of dentists signed Flagg's manifesto, and the wild statements put around by his opponents did Morton's cause incalculable damage. The movement against him gathered momentum and might easily have forced doctors to give up the use of ether. "To overcome their prejudice and suspicion which they have thrown upon the use of the inhaling vapour," Morton said, "requires all my logic and much time."[9]

Fortunately he had the support of men like Warren and Bigelow, who were prepared to face all sorts of opposition to continue with what was so clearly a discovery of enormous benefit to mankind. They might have replied to the critics as Simpson did a few years later, when Dr Montgomery, the head of the School of Midwifery in Dublin, said: "I do not believe that anyone in Dublin has as yet used ether in midwifery; the feeling is very strong against its use in ordinary cases, and merely to avert the ordinary amount of pain which the Almighty has seen fit—and most wisely we cannot doubt—to allot to natural labour, and in this feeling I heartily and entirely concur." Simpson retorted: "I do not believe that anyone in Dublin has as yet used a carriage in locomotion; the feeling is very strong against its use in ordinary progress, and merely to avert the ordinary amount of fatigue which the Almighty has seen fit—and most wisely we cannot doubt—to allot to natural walking, and in this feeling I heartily and entirely concur!"[10]

Above all it was a victory for common sense. Faced with the alternative of using ether or suffering, patients saw no compelling reason to be subjected to intolerable pain. A description of a contemporary operation leaves no doubt to how one patient felt. A respectable farmer had divided one of the arteries in the palm of his hand in an accident, and when it proved impossible to stop the bleeding the doctors decided to tie the artery. They told the farmer they would give him something to prevent the pain, but his wife called them aside and said that her husband, after a conversation with her, had decided not to inhale the ether, the reason being that they both considered it wrong; she added that, having fortified himself by prayer, he felt himself sufficiently prepared, and would not endeavour to escape any of that punishment which had been ordained man for his sin.

Preparations were begun, and with a last kiss his wife left the room to go and pray again that his resolution might be further strengthened. The man's hand was placed in position upon a table, and the surgeon, with one clean, quick cut, divided the skin immediately over the artery. But the good farmer was hardly as much fortified as he supposed, for "with a terrific yell, which could have been heard almost as far as a steam whistle, he broke from the hands which endeavoured to restrain him, and ordered them to stop".

"Phew!" said he. "That was awful. Why, Doctor, I didn't know it was to hurt like that."

"Certainly," said Dr Wyman, "I told you it would pain some. How do you expect any cutting can be done and you not feel it? Come, my good friend, sit down and let me finish, it will soon be through."

"But wait, is it going to hurt like that all the rest of the time?" Wyman had to struggle to keep a straight face and said, it would in some degree, but not nearly as much.

"Yes, Doctor, but I can't stand it; you say that the stuff you have in that little bottle will keep me from feeling it? You do? Well now, Doctor, do you think it would be really wrong to take it? Say just a little enough to keep off the worst of the pain, but still let me feel some—of course you don't. You are a good man, Doctor, and you wouldn't do anything wrong I know; besides, if you recommend it to me, the blame ought to fall upon you." After pausing a minute in deep agitation he suddenly brought his huge fist with a loud thump upon the table, and with a preliminary specimen of "muscular English" exclaimed, "Well, wicked or not, Doctor, I guess I'll go the ether!"[11]

While repudiating the vicious attacks made upon him Morton was still busy perfecting his method. He had now given up his medical studies to administer ether for the operations performed at the hospital. He was also busy writing pamphlets explaining the technique involved, and published a weekly circular describing his experiments. Later he included articles and letters which came from all over America giving details of operations and testifying to the successful use of ether. Altogether five editions were issued under Morton's supervision, and he attempted to make a synopsis of the information he had gleaned. It was these pamphlets, Bigelow's paper, and Morton's booklet *On the Proper Mode of Administering Sulphuric Ether by Inhalation* which provided the basic information on which an enormous body of literature has since been built. Morton also spent a lot of his time answering the letters which poured in from all over the world asking for further information. Certainly no one could have worked harder or more selflessly than Morton, but it was a long-drawn-out battle, fought on many fronts at the same time, and one which constantly sapped his strength and energy.

Morton's name was now on everyone's lips. All of Boston knew of his momentous discovery and of the marvellous operations at the hospital. The newspapers were full of praise, and the congratulations were pouring in. But with the admiration came envy and jealousy, for, as Francis Bacon said: "So long as a thing has not been achieved, people are surprised when they are told it is possible; but as soon as it has taken place, they wonder why no one thought of it before." As the success of Morton's discovery became more and more assured there appeared everywhere what the editor of *The Lancet* was to describe as "the large class of jump-up-behinders". One of these was Professor Charles Jackson.

When Jackson had first heard of Morton's discovery he had refused absolutely to give Morton a certificate for its use, and went round telling everyone that ether was not as harmless as they imagined. For some time he had refused to have anything to do with the patent because he was afraid something might go wrong and patients would be killed. Even when ether proved to be safe he still hesitated to take part in case some scandal about the patent endangered his professional standing. But when the operations proved successful Jackson changed his tune. When the doctors hailed Morton's discovery as the greatest of the century and likely to secure fame and fortune for its inventor Jackson began to think again.

He was an ambitious man. He easily persuaded himself that Morton was nothing but a pushing, uneducated dentist who could never have made a discovery on his own, and asked himself why Morton should have all the honour and glory, and collect a fortune too, while he, Jackson, who had given him so much advice, was fobbed off with a mere 10 per cent? Had he not been tricked in the same way by Morse, a mere portrait painter—and Beaumont and Schönbein? In his half-mad mind truth and desires easily became mixed, and this time he determined not to let a little dentist get away with a discovery which would resound round the world and make a fortune.

When Jackson went to Warren's house for a meeting of the Thursday Evening Club he told Warren that he himself had first suggested the preparation to Morton. Warren was more than surprised at such a claim, for from his own personal knowledge of the affair he was well aware that Jackson had taken no part, and that, in fact, he had never even attended an operation at which the preparation had been administered. No doubt Jackson was not the first to make such a claim, but as the contents were still secret at that time Warren wrote to him the following day to inquire the nature of Morton's preparation. Jackson did not answer, and even when Warren asked him on a future occasion he again declined to enlighten Warren, saying it was against the spirit of his arrangement with Morton. On October 29th Warren once more wrote to Jackson to ask him to administer the preparation at an operation, but it was quite clear that Jackson was not capable of doing so, for he pleaded that he was off on some geological expedition and could not come.

After the operation on Alice Mohan had proved the discovery a great success, and after the Letters of Patent had been formally granted on November 12th, Jackson stepped up his campaign. Hearing that Jackson was connected with the patent, Bigelow when he was writing his paper describing the new discovery and the operations at the hospital went round to see Jackson. Jackson was out, and Bigelow left a message with

Mrs Jackson for her husband to meet him at Dr Gould's house on the following Sunday evening, the 15th of November, 1846. On the Saturday, the 14th of November, Eddy was very surprised to receive a visit from Hayes, of Loring and Hayes, Jackson's lawyers, who had come to try to get Jackson a better percentage of the profits of the patent. Eddy was very upset that Jackson had not come personally, but had sent his lawyer to act for him instead, and so went round to call on Jackson himself the following afternoon, the 15th of November.

Eddy found Dr and Mrs Jackson in the rear parlour. Jackson was in a most excited state. "I claim the whole of it, it is mine!" he kept on shouting. "He did nothing but under my prescription!"[12] Eddy begged him to keep calm and not to make a claim that could not possibly be substantiated, but later that evening, when Bigelow, Morton, and Eddy had all assembled at Gould's house as arranged, Jackson suddenly burst in "declaiming vociferously". He quietened down a little when Bigelow showed him his paper, and appeared to be mollified when Bigelow agreed to alter his statement to read simply that "the patent bears the name of Charles T. Jackson, a distinguished chemist, and of Dr Morton, a skilled dentist of this city, as inventors, and has been issued to the latter gentleman as proprietor".[13]

When they began to discuss the matter Jackson again kept on insisting that he should be given the credit for the discovery. Again he showed signs of great agitation and began to make wild claims. Morton was amazed. He had heard rumours of this sort of talk, but it was so far from the truth that he could still not believe his ears. How could Jackson make such outrageous claims in front of these people who knew so well what had happened? Ether had been used in medicine for years, but everyone including Jackson had failed to realize its potentialities. They all knew perfectly well that it was Morton's idea, that he was the one who had done all the experiments, and that he alone had borne the responsibility of carrying it through to a successful conclusion. They all knew that Jackson had taken no part in the operations, and that, in fact, his name had not even been mentioned until afterwards.

Eddy begged Jackson to calm down, and pressed them both to reconcile their claims. Morton was polite, but made no secret of his feelings. Gould pleaded with them to try to understand each other's point of view, and said he was glad to see them both face to face, for he knew that if Jackson stated his claims fully Morton would admit them. In fact Morton—magnanimous as usual—did concede several points. He admitted that Jackson's advice on the use of sulphuric instead of chloric ether had been of great help to him and had saved him time on further experiments.

In spite of Morton's attempts to come to some agreement, Jackson continued to insist that it had been he who had been responsible. Again there was an uproar as Jackson insisted that he could prove this, while Morton

108

begged leave to doubt his statements. Eventually, after he had been forced to admit that in fact he had never tried at all to etherize a patient for an operation, Jackson climbed down and agreed to accept the advice of the others present. Converted, it seemed, with Morton's permission he agreed to be described as having had some part in the discovery. Morton had conceded a great deal, and it appeared to everyone there that the matter was now finally settled. But it showed how little they knew of Jackson's mentality, for what he failed to get one way he simply set about trying to get in another.

On the way home with Eddy Jackson again returned to the business side of the patent. Under the terms of their agreement Eddy was to receive 25 per cent of the proceeds for handling the patent, Jackson 10 per cent, and Morton 65. Jackson now proposed that he should have 10 per cent of Morton's and Eddy's share too, for he was quite convinced that the patent was going to make a lot of money, and he was determined to get as much as he possibly could for himself. Eddy did not see why he should give up any of his share to Jackson, and, in fact, thought he had managed to talk Jackson out of the idea. But he was wrong, for the following day Jackson came to see Eddy, accompanied now by his lawyer Hayes. This time they both threatened Eddy that unless he met Jackson's demand for an increased percentage Jackson would "make communications abroad" which would ruin both him and Morton. They insisted, moreover, that Eddy must agree to settle with them before the British mailboat sailed that day for Liverpool.

Eddy's father, Caleb Eddy, was furious. He was disgusted that Jackson —an old and trusted friend of his—should behave in this way, and was quick to tell him so. Hayes then produced a new agreement he had brought with him which gave terms differing considerably from those already agreed. Eddy was even more furious than his father at these manœuvres and at Jackson's attempts at blackmail, and refused to have anything to do with such an agreement. He was completely at a loss to understand how someone like Jackson—a reputable scientist, a Christian gentleman, highly respected in the town, and, above all, a great family friend of his—could act like this. Jackson seemed a changed man, and, indeed, he was. What in the case of Beaumont and Morse had been only the first signs of madness had now developed and deepened into paranoia. But although the subject began to dominate him, he still used his brilliant brain to full effect, devoting it now to devising his cunning schemes.

So, unsuccessful in his attempt to blackmail Eddy, he again pretended to back down with sweet reasonableness. Although only a cloak for even more treacherous behaviour, his attitude completely disarmed Bigelow, Gould, and all the others who would have leapt to Morton's defence had they but known Jackson's real intentions. Failing entirely to understand Jackson and his terrible thirst for fame, they were completely taken in by his charm. Fooled by his apparently submissive behaviour, they accepted his word that he had now dropped his claim and believed that he had made a genuine mistake in supposing that he had taken a larger part in the discovery than they knew to be the case. Now that he was prepared to withdraw and Morton to forgive him, they were anxious to consider the matter closed, but little did they realize that their opposition to his plans had served only to persuade him to resort to even more dishonest and deceitful methods, as like a child he sought now to gain his ends by guile.

The United States at that time was still small and insignificant compared with the older countries, and Jackson knew that if he wanted world acclaim it was to Europe he must look, not to the United States. And in Europe he had many friends. After graduating in America Jackson had spent a year studying in Paris among mineralogists and scientists, many of whom were now in very influential positions. Telling no one what he was going to do, he sat down and wrote a letter to one of them, Élie de Beaumont, Professor of Geology in Paris and a very important member of the French Academy of Sciences. Jackson, of course, at that time had not even seen a painless operation, but that did not deter him at all from writing to Beaumont on the subject, for his sinister scheme depended upon his letter reaching Beaumont as quickly as possible. If he were to succeed at all it must go by the mailboat leaving immediately for Europe. Hurriedly he wrote the letter and put a sealed statement inside and sent it off. Meanwhile he told no one what he had done. No one knew that he had written to Beaumont on the subject, least of all Morton. Quite oblivious of the time bomb which Jackson had so skilfully placed beneath him, Morton continued with his hard work.

NOTES TO CHAPTER X

1. *The Lancet,* I, 1847.
2. *Ibid.*
3. Nathan Rice, *Trials of a Public Benefactor.*
4. *Ibid.*
5. *Ibid.*
6. *Ibid.*
7. *Ibid.*
8. *McClure's Magazine,* September 1896.
9. Nathan Rice, *op. cit.*
10. James Simpson, *Landmarks in the Struggle between Science and Religion.*
11. Nathan Rice, *op. cit.*
12. *Ibid.*
13. *The Lancet, op. cit.*

CHAPTER

XI

S O far his discovery had been given no proper name, and was referred to merely as "Morton's preparation", "the gas", "the mixture", or some such term. Now that it was to be used throughout the world Morton's friends insisted that what had been described as a "gift from Heaven", "the most God-like discovery of this or any other age", should have an appropriate name. Attempts were made to find one which would match the magnitude of the discovery, and Morton and some of his friends gathered at Gould's house on November 20th, 1846, to discuss the latest developments and to find a good name for it. Gould read out a long list which had so far been suggested, one of which was 'letheon', from the river Lethe of Greek mythology, a draught of whose waters expunged all painful memories of past life. When it was read out Morton jumped up excitedly and exclaimed that there could surely be no better name than this. Everyone there agreed, except for Oliver Wendell Holmes. Holmes was a professor of anatomy at Harvard, founder of the *Atlantic Monthly* magazine, and a well-known poet; in fact, it was from one of his poems that Mark Twain unconsciously stole the dedication for his *Innocents Abroad*. Holmes was not satisfied with the name 'letheon', and thought that in such an age of science Morton should find one which would have more meaning scientifically. He promised to see what he could devise, and the following day, November 21st, 1846, he wrote to Morton:

DEAR SIR,
  Everyone wants to have a hand in a great discovery. All I do is to give a hint or two, as to names. . . .
  The state should I think be called 'Anaesthesia'. . . . The adjective will be 'Anaesthetic'. . . .
  I would have a name pretty soon, and consult some accomplished

111

scholar, such as President Everett or Dr Bigelow senior, before fixing upon the terms, which will be repeated by the tongue of every civilised race of mankind. . . .

Respectfully yours,
OLIVER WENDELL HOLMES.[1]

At first the name 'letheon' was used, but later, impressed with Holmes's suggestion and with the further advice of Everett and Jacob Bigelow, Morton adopted the name 'anaesthesia'. Applied now generally with all such drugs, as Holmes so correctly prophesied, the term has been repeated by the "tongue of every civilised race of mankind". That Morton's name has not been coupled with it has been a disgrace, but hardly had his success become known when Morton's hour of glory turned to one of tragedy. Jackson was now openly boasting that he had given Morton the idea for his discovery, but offered no evidence to support his claim. Morton was much too preoccupied with the introduction of anaesthesia to treat him seriously, and with so much to be done—writing pamphlets, organizing the manufacture of the inhalers, answering the vast correspondence, besides administering the ether for the operations carried out at the hospital—there was little time for much else. Only someone of Morton's energy and dedication could have achieved so much, for, as his lawyer said, he "hardly knew a full night's rest or a regular meal, for three months". He should have been buoyed up by his great and resounding success, but he seems throughout this time, although still unaware of Jackson's treachery, to have sensed that there was a terrible time ahead.

While Morton was perfecting his method for securing anaesthesia Jackson was busy with his own plans. On November 21st, 1846, he attended an operation at Bromfield House, the private wing of the hospital, the first operation that Jackson had ever seen performed under anaesthetic. Morton administered the ether, and Warren's son, Mason Warren, operated. John Collins Warren noticed Jackson among the spectators, but he took no part at all in the operation. Jackson was not yet prepared to show his hand, but all the time he was quietly and methodically laying the foundation for his cunning plot, watching carefully all that Morton and the doctors were doing, quietly noting the effects of the anaesthetic, and studying its implications.

Morton's patent seemed secure, and he went rapidly ahead with his grandiose plans, sending inhalers and full instructions to the hospitals, and personal models to the crowned heads of Europe—King Louis-Philippe of France, King Leopold of the Belgians, King Charles of Sweden, Tsar Nicholas of Russia, the Emperor Ferdinand of Austria, King Ernest of Hanover, King William of Holland, Christian VIII of Denmark, Frederick of Saxony, Louis of Bavaria, even Charles Albert, King of Sardinia. He also sent his apparatus to all the distinguished surgeons, and soon there was hardly a hospital in America, a ruler in Europe, or a surgeon or

112

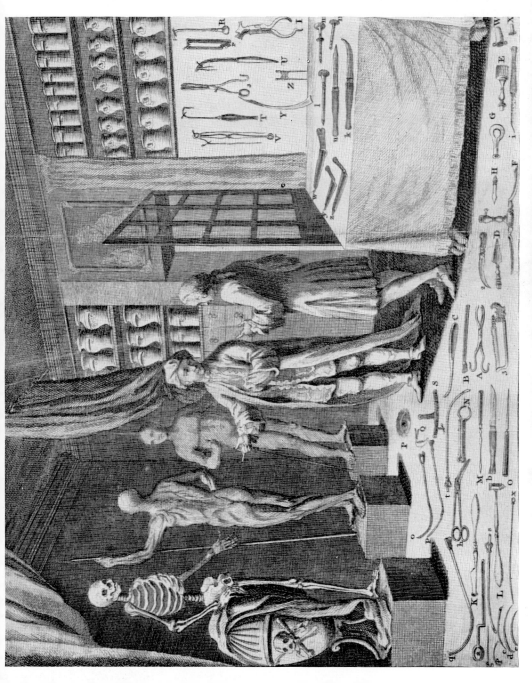

An early surgery,
with instruments

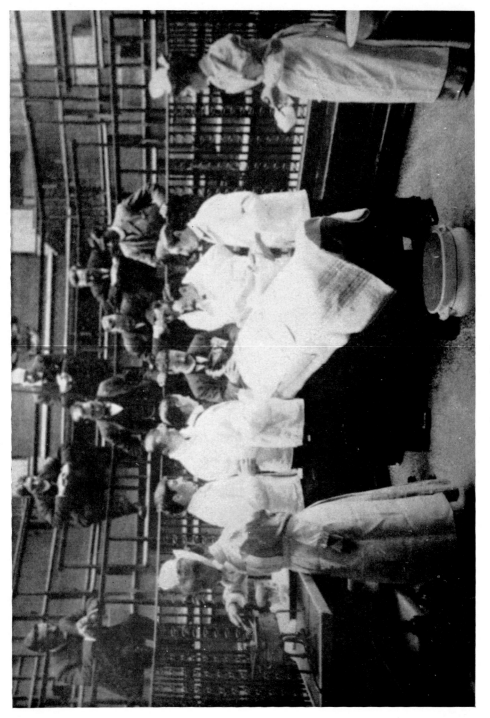

An operating theatre of 1898

scientist of any note who had not received one of Morton's inhalers. His agents were leaving for the far corners of the world to secure the patent right, and copies of Bigelow's paper had been sent off on the steamer leaving for Europe.

When Jackson got wind of these activities he was appalled. Previously Morton had confined his attentions to America, but now, by extending his interests to Europe, Jackson was afraid Morton was going to ruin his brilliant scheme. The most devastating news of all was that Morton had sent off an inhaler to Dr Willis Fisher in Paris, and it was this that forced Jackson's hand. Straight away, on December 1st, he wrote a letter to Élie de Beaumont to ask him to open the sealed statement he had sent previously, and to communicate its contents at once to the great French Academy of Sciences.

But Paris was not his only target. Jackson did not forget his other influential friends and acquaintances, and wrote to the leading scientists and intellectuals, men like Von Humboldt. Alexander von Humboldt was a Prussian, generally regarded as one of the greatest scientists of the day, a friend of King Frederick William IV and of King Louis-Philippe. Von Humboldt had just made a profound impression with the first volume of his *Kosmos*, both in the European academies and in the Court circles. He must know of Jackson, and as a fellow-geologist would surely accept his statement.

Mail to Europe then took about two weeks or so, for telegraphic communication had not yet been established and the new steamboats were not much quicker than the sailing-ships which still plied with them. Often the steamboats carried some sail themselves to take advantage of the wind and save some of the enormous amounts of coal which their engines needed. Having written all his letters, Jackson sat back to wait, secure in the knowledge that soon all Europe would ring with the name of Professor Charles T. Jackson.

But if Jackson was the most cunning and stealthy of Morton's opponents he was by no means the only one. As Milton said:

> The invention all admired, and each how he
> To be the inventor missed, so easy it seemed
> Once found, which yet unfound most would have thought
> Impossible.

While Jackson was going quietly to work Horace Wells strode into action in his usual impetuous fashion. Morton's marvellous success became known just as Wells was about to leave for France. His Scientific Panorama at Hartford had closed and he felt annoyed that Morton had succeeded where he had so dismally failed. He had always believed that he could have achieved marvellous results with his laughing gas if he had only been given the chance, and the thought that Morton had pressed on

113

to success and looked like making a fortune out of it rankled deeply with him. If ether was effective, so was laughing gas, he told himself, and if only his demonstration at the hospital had not failed it would have been he and not Morton who was being acclaimed throughout the world. He found it easy to convince himself that he should have the honour, not Morton, nor Jackson either, and impetuously he wrote off to the *Hartford Courant*. His letter was published on December 7th: "As Dr Charles T. Jackson and W. T. G. Morton claim to be the originators of this invaluable discovery, I will give a short history of its introduction, that the public may decide to whom belongs the honour. . . . When I was deciding what exhilarating agent to use, it immediately occurred to me that it would be best to use nitrous oxide gas, or sulphuric ether. I advised with Dr Marcy, of this city, and by his advice I continued to use the former. . . . If Dr Jackson and Morton claim that they use something else, I reply that it is the same in principle if not in name."

This was obviously ridiculous. Wells had given up all hopes of achieving painless extractions two years before, and but for Morton's hard work the whole thing would have ended there. His claim that laughing gas had the same effect as ether was clearly nonsense, for by itself nitrous oxide can never give the sure, steady anaesthesia necessary for surgical operations, and it was many more years before it was used even for extracting teeth. Anyway, Wells himself did not appear to treat his claim very seriously, for the day after writing the letter he set out for France to buy engravings. Obviously his first reaction, like Jackson's, had been to underestimate the importance of Morton's discovery, and having made a feeble attempt to claim the honour of discovering anaesthesia, he again abandoned the subject.

Jackson, on the other hand, was now fully aware of the momentous nature of the discovery, and, secure in the knowledge that his statement was already in the hands of the French Academy of Sciences, began to press Morton to accept his claim. He knew Morton was being attacked from all sides, and thought he would be so glad of his support that he would be prepared to pay a price for it. On January 28th, 1847, he therefore got his lawyers, Loring and Hayes, to write Morton a letter demanding that Jackson should be given 25 per cent of all returns from the patent, instead of the 10 per cent previously agreed. "Ten per cent . . . is altogether inadequate," they wrote. "Dr Jackson must be considered as deserving something more than double that commission for his interest in a discovery from which both of you (Morton and Eddy) have profited and will continue to profit so much."[2]

In fact, neither Morton nor Eddy had made any profit from the patent so far, for there had been many expenses but very little return. The lawyers went on to point out that Morton would need Jackson's support to make sure that the patent was upheld, so that they could all make the

114

"expected large sums" out of it. They made it clear that an increase in Jackson's share was the price of his collaboration with Morton, and said: "A sense of what is generous and honourable (not to say anything of the justice of any further claim) should influence you in deciding to give Dr Jackson, not a paltry percentage, but what may be considered a fair share of the profits. . . . We think the least that, in justice to yourselves and Dr Jackson, you can offer, is 20 per cent of the profits . . . both at home and abroad, in settlement of his claims upon you."[8]

The lawyers begged Morton to make the dispute between himself and Jackson "as little public as possible", obviously hoping to persuade Morton not to enlist popular support until Jackson had time to marshal his own forces and to get the backing of all his eminent European friends. Morton was outraged at Jackson's behaviour. Jackson had not made the discovery, had taken none of the vast responsibility for trying it out on patients, and was still doing nothing to help with its development. At first he had asked for a fee of 500 dollars for the information. Then he was content to settle for 10 per cent of the patent. Now he was trying to get twenty-five. Morton could see that all Jackson wanted was to grab as much as he could. He knew that his demand was most unjust, and he absolutely refused to have anything to do with it. Jackson was furious at Morton's reaction, but consoled himself with gloating at the thought of what was happening in Europe. Jackson was not the only one expecting news. Morton too was waiting eagerly to hear the effect of his discovery upon the great medical and scientific men of Europe. He imagined the incredulity of these grand figures at the discovery of a little American dentist. He pictured the excitement of the first painless operations in Europe. He was certain that his discovery would be an immediate sensation and that his name would be on everyone's lips. Then, he told his wife and friends, would all his work, all his experiments, all his sacrifices, have been worth while. Paris, London, Vienna, Berlin—the whole wide world would be talking about him. He could barely think of anything else as he waited impatiently each day for the return mail from Europe and the report that Edward Warren had promised to send him.

When at long last the letter came Morton excitedly tore it open. At first, Edward Warren reported, all had gone well. The operations carried out under ether had been a great success, and everyone was wildly enthusiastic. When Wells had turned up in Paris and had declared he had been the first with laughing gas some had been impressed with his claim. But Wells was rather a figure of fun, and not too much attention was paid to him. Then the matter had come before the French Academy of Sciences, the greatest scientific body in France, and, indeed, perhaps in the world at that time. All of France was talking about the marvellous new painless surgery, and when the Academy met again on Monday, January 18th, 1847, to discuss the discovery of anaesthesia the leading authorities

115

were there—Velpeau, Serres, and Roux, everyone—all anxious to hear the details of this great new discovery. But then a shocking thing had happened for, instead of the universal acclamation of Morton's work that Warren had expected, Élie de Beaumont had got to his feet and read out to the meeting a long statement from Dr Charles T. Jackson. It began: "I ask leave to communicate through you to the Academy of Sciences a discovery which I have made. . . . I have lately put it to use, by persuading a dentist of this city to administer the vapour of ether to persons from whom he was to extract teeth. . . . I then requested this dentist to go to the Massachusetts General Hospital and administer the vapour of ether to a patient about to undergo a painful surgical operation. . . ."[4]

Morton was absolutely astounded when he read this. How could Jackson possibly pretend it was his discovery? How could Jackson possibly say he was only a hireling? Morton could hardly believe his eyes, for Jackson's letter was dated November 13th, the day after the patent was granted, and at that time he had never even seen an operation with ether! But this did not bother Jackson. To try to prove that he had been experimenting before Morton he described the experiments he said he had made himself with sulphuric ether some five or six years before, claiming that he had stumbled upon the discovery after having inhaled a quantity of chlorine gas. Suddenly Morton could see it all, and how Jackson had made up his statement, for in Pereira's *Elements of Materia Medica*, the book which had so encouraged him in his own experiments, Morton recalled the passage: "The vapour of ether inhaled . . . to relieve the effect caused by the *accidental inhalation of chlorine gas* [author's italics]."

Not for nothing was Jackson a trained scientist, and his statement was an expert scientific report, with everything put in a scholarly fashion likely to appeal to the learned gentlemen of the Academy of Sciences and with a full description of the method of administration of the ether and its effects. Morton was appalled. But he could see too how clever Jackson had been. When he had written his letter on November 13th, 1846, he had never in his life administered ether for a surgical operation—or even at that time seen it done. Morton, on the other hand, had already administered the anaesthetic for many important operations, watched publicly by hundreds of people. His position in Boston was almost unassailable, and Jackson knew that his only hope of wresting the honour from him was to marshal his friends in Europe and to try to win the decision there. He knew he must act fast to establish his claim to Morton's discovery, and that his letter had to be sent off on the mailboat leaving at once for Europe.

But Jackson was cautious as well as sly. When he wrote his statement at the beginning of November he was still not really convinced that Morton's discovery was absolutely safe. If it did turn out to be dangerous in general use, or even ineffective, his statement would have made him look a fool in the eyes of all his important European friends. He dare not

116

risk this, and so had thought up a very clever scheme. This was to seal his statement claiming to have discovered anaesthesia and to send it with a covering letter, telling Beaumont not to open it until he sent him further directions. If anything had gone wrong, he could have written immediately to Beaumont to ask him to destroy his statement unopened and unread. No one would then have known that Jackson had claimed to be responsible for introducing anaesthesia. No one would then have known that Jackson had blundered and made a fool of himself.

Meantime neither Morton nor Bigelow nor Warren nor anyone else in Boston who knew the real facts of the discovery, had any inkling of what Jackson was doing. It was certainly an artful move. When, as actually happened, ether did prove a success—and the moment Jackson heard that copies of Bigelow's paper were being sent to Europe and that Morton was sending details of his discovery and inhalers to all the leading scientists and crowned heads of Europe—he had written off to Beaumont to ask him to open his statement and place it before the Academy of Sciences. While Morton and Bigelow had waited until they were able to say it was completely safe, Jackson had rushed in to steal the honour and glory for himself.

Obviously the claim had no more truth than all his other attempts—to steal Morse's electric telegraph, to take the credit for William Beaumont's experiments on St Martin, or to claim Schönbein's discovery of guncotton. If he had really made this momentous discovery five years before, why had he said nothing until after Morton made his discovery public? Surely he would at least have mentioned it to Warren—a colleague and an old friend of his? Yet Warren testified later that: "I hereby declare and certify to the best of my knowledge and recollection, that I have never heard of the use of sulphuric ether, by inhalation, as a means of preventing the pain of surgical operations, until it was suggested by William T. G. Morton in the latter part of October 1846."[5]

Jackson's statement was clearly all lies, for if he had really found the means to prevent pain five years before, why did he leave humanity to go on suffering such agonies for all these long years? When his aunt visited Morton in 1844 and remained several hours in the dental chair begging for something to make her insensible, Jackson was present, but made no suggestion of anything to produce insensibility. Dr Jacob Bigelow, Henry's father, made the position quite plain when he said: "If Dr Jackson did make his discovery in 1842, he stands accountable for the mass of human misery which he has permitted his fellow creatures to undergo from the time when he made his discovery, to the time when Dr Morton made his. In charity we prefer to believe that up to the latter period Dr Jackson had no definite notion of the real power of ether in surgery."[6]

If, too, the discovery had really been Jackson's, as he said, why did he not come to any of the operations? For a man in Jackson's position to have gone away and left an unqualified dentist to administer dangerous new drugs on his own would have been totally irresponsible, reprehensible, and, indeed, quite, unbelievable.

Again, if he had been the real discoverer, would Jackson have accepted only 10 per cent of the patent when he was in a position to demand the whole? But in spite of all this, in spite of the fact that his statement to the French Academy was unsupported, while hundreds of people had watched Morton publicly administer the anaesthetic, Jackson's plot was obviously very clever.

The letter (in French), written on November 13th, 1846, and in the hands of the Academy since December 28th, was among the earliest information about the discovery to have been received in France. It requested: "I should be deeply grateful if the Academy of Sciences would have the goodness to appoint a commission to prove the correctness of the assertions which I have made to you on the marvellous effects of the inhalation of sulphuric ether."[7]

It was an artful move to suggest that they should appoint a commission. Jackson had spent a year in Paris on post-graduate study and had made many friends who were now in influential positions. He knew that if Paris accepted him as the discoverer the rest of the scientific world would most probably follow suit. Professor de Beaumont was a great friend of his and a powerful figure in the Academy. In fact, he was made its Permanent Secretary soon after, and when the matter came up at the meeting on January 18th, 1847, the members were very impressed by his words about his old colleague Jackson. Had it not been for Velpeau, who said he had heard about the new discovery from Willis Fisher, there would have been no mention of Morton's name at all. Velpeau described the new method, but said that of course he had not realized that Morton was only a dentist —a hireling acting under Professor Jackson's orders. Poor Morton, it seemed as if Jackson had established himself as the discoverer. Roux, Serres, everyone, they were all apparently convinced that it was the eminent Boston scientist Professor Charles Jackson, and ordered a record to this effect to be made in the minutes. The Academy went on to appoint a special commission, just as Jackson had asked, to report on anaesthesia and honour its discoverer, Professor Charles Jackson.

When Morton heard this devastating news he realized how weak his own position was. The members of the Academy would never have heard of him, a small-town dentist, with no education, no degrees or diplomas, and no reputation. He would hardly cut much of a figure before the learned members, all of whom had honours and medals and doctorates from old and famous European universities. He had no experience of such affairs and would find it difficult to argue his case in scientific terms in French before such an august body. He was in despair. Bitterly he reflected that Jackson had written his second letter just after he had personally assured Bigelow, Gould, Eddy, and the others that he was quite satisfied to be named as co-discoverer. After coming to an agreement with them he had immediately sat down and written this statement, all behind their backs. How despicable! Poor Morton, after all his years of hard work and patient experimenting, after all his sacrifice, instead of hearing that he had been acclaimed in Europe, it was Jackson who had been honoured. He was heartbroken.

But what could be done? Edward Warren had said that Professor de Beaumont seemed already to have gained the day for Jackson. Beaumont was one of their most influential members. He had personally asserted that the eminent Professor Jackson of Boston was the discoverer, and the Academy had accepted his word without question. It would be difficult now to get the Academy to change its declared view, and Warren implored Morton to take immediate steps to safeguard his own position and to protect his patent rights; otherwise there would be nothing anyone could do to retrieve the position.

To Morton there was only one thing to do. He must go and see Jackson at once and confront him with Warren's letter. He must insist on Jackson's issuing a retraction immediately. If necessary, he would start proceedings to protect his name, for Jackson was just trying the same trick he had played upon Morse, and Morton was determined to see that he did not get away with it.

Jackson was in his laboratory when Morton burst in on him furiously and began to rage at him. How dare he try to steal his discovery! How dare he write the letter to Beaumont behind his back! He stormed round the laboratory, waving Warren's letter in Jackson's face, saying all Boston knew that his statement was just a pack of lies, and that he would force him to issue an immediate disclaimer, or otherwise he would sue him.

Jackson took it all quite calmly, and as usual, when he was confronted with his own misdeeds, appeared to be most apologetic and utterly disarming. He explained that there must have been some silly mistake, and that no doubt his old friend Beaumont had misunderstood, and for the sake of friendship overstated, the part he had played in the discovery. He offered to write at once to tell Beaumont the truth of the matter, and to set it right with the Academy of Sciences by assuring them that Morton was the real discoverer.

No one could be more disarming or more conciliatory than Jackson when he wanted to, and he readily persuaded Morton to accept his word as a gentleman that he would soon put matters right. Like many mad people, at his most dangerous Jackson appeared frank and charming and absolutely sincere in what he said. He seemed able to persuade people to accept his statements as honest and his intentions as genuine, and men more educated in the ways of the world than Morton were completely taken in.

119

So, accepting Jackson's word, Morton apologized for his hasty behaviour and left. Mollified, he went home to wait for Jackson to establish once and for all the truth that it was really his discovery. In this event Morton was to be terribly disappointed.

NOTES TO CHAPTER XI

1. Nathan Rice, *Trials of a Public Benefactor*.
2. *Ibid.*
3. *Ibid.*
4. Académie des Sciences, C. R., 1847, 24.
5. Nathan Rice, *op. cit.*
6. *Ibid.*
7. Académie des Sciences, *op. cit.*

CHAPTER

XII

ORTON was now fighting on all fronts. Rival dentists were becoming more and more jealous of him and his patent, and Dr Josiah Flagg's Committee of Vigilance had succeeded in collecting hundreds of signatures for the manifesto condemning the new practice. In fact, the opposition to the use of ether, or perhaps to paying the licence fee for it, became so formidable that Keep, who was to have used Morton's preparation for painless extractions, thought it prudent to withdraw from his partnership with Morton. Their agreement, signed on November 28th, 1846, was to have lasted for ten years, but actually was terminated after a little more than a month. They parted quite amicably, for Morton always tried to remain on the best of terms with everyone and to assure Keep that he bore him no ill-will he sent him a handsome parting present of a gold pen and pencil.

Arguments still raged also in the medical world on the merits of anaesthesia. Diehards continued to reject the new method, and in spite of all Morton's efforts to promote it, painless surgery continued to be resisted by many doctors, and even by some of the hospitals. A Professor Mütter of Philadelphia declared that he did not consider anything worth using which "unquestionably subjects the patient to the risk of losing his life", and even in November 1847 the *Annual Report on Surgery*, read before the College of Physicians in Pennsylvania by Dr Isaac Paris, stated: "At the Pennsylvania Hospital in this city it has not been tried at all, being considered by the judicious surgeons of that institution as a remedy of doubtful safety."[1]

In 1846 the United States went to war with Mexico, and Morton wrote offering to supply inhalers to the Army at wholesale prices and to instruct the Army surgeons in their use. Surely nowhere could the benefits of anaesthesia be more urgently needed than in relieving the terrible agonies of soldiers wounded in battle, but even here Morton's discovery was to be rejected. On May 3rd, 1847, the Surgeon-General replied to Morton's offer:

It is believed that the highly volatile character itself is ill-adapted to the rough usage it would necessarily encounter on the field of battle.

For this and other reasons, which it is unnecessary now to detail, I must decline to recommend the use of your remedy in the surgical operations of the Army.

Very respectfully,
Your obedient Servant.[2]

The Secretary of the Navy also wrote, on April 17th, 1847:

The Chief of that Bureau [of Medicine and Surgery] reports that the article may be of some service for the use of large hospitals, but does not think it expedient for the Department to incur any expense for its introduction to the general service, in which opinion the Department concurs.[3]

It is difficult to imagine more heartless and typically bureaucratic letters, rejecting out of hand an attempt to alleviate the terrible sufferings of the wounded, simply because of the trouble and expense involved, and Morton was disgusted at their response. He redoubled his efforts to promote anaesthesia—publicizing his method, circulating his magazine as widely as possible, arranging for the manufacture of inhalers, and training operators to administer the ether.

While Morton was slaving away Jackson continued his campaign. At last, on January 2nd, 1847, he officially attended an operation at the hospital, and arrived carrying bags of oxygen which he said might be useful in the event of asphyxia. But here he betrayed his complete ignorance of the experience gained since the days of the first operations, for both Bigelow and Morton were now well aware that sufficient atmospheric air was essential and had taken steps to ensure this by removing the inhaler valves. Jackson continued to play a very clever game, and both to establish his claim with Morton and also to defend his position against any of the other contenders. On January 7th, 1847, he wrote to Warren:

I am now glad that I have secured the discovery by law, for the pretenders will have to test their claims thereby. I did not wish to be troubled with the business matters pertaining to the sale of patent rights, and so I assigned to Mr Morton my right in the patent, he agreeing to take charge of the business and to pay me 10 per cent as my proportion of the sales of licences. I think Mr Wells is endeavouring to make a disturbance for the sake of notoriety, for he cannot suppose he can show the least claim to the discovery.[4]

Everywhere he went he spread lies about Morton. He had written to

122

Paris to Josiah Dwight Whitney, one of the first great American geologists, then just starting his career: "Morton and Eddy are in co-partnership, and are making money out of my invention, and even refuse me a paltry sum of 10 per cent on net profits of sales in Europe. Eddy tendered me an offer of 5 per cent, and Morton declined paying me a cent."[5] In fact, as Jackson knew very well, there had been no profits so far. At that time Boston was still quite a small town, and among the few professional men Jackson's attitude had created a very tense and difficult situation. Eventually it became so embarrassing that a committee of doctors from the hospital called on him to protest at the statements he had been making about Morton. Jackson seemed unabashed, saying that there must, of course, have been some misunderstanding but promising to make amends.

As word of all this got round to Morton he became more and more disheartened, and began to doubt whether Jackson was going to do anything to see that Beaumont knew the facts, or even that he had ever intended to do so. Since their last stormy meeting over the news from Beaumont Jackson had merely pressed his claim for a bigger share of the patent revenues, and in the last week of February 1847 he sent his lawyer to open negotiations with Morton for a settlement of his grievances. They had frequent discussions throughout the week, and all the time the lawyer proclaimed Jackson's sincerest regret at the misunderstanding which had arisen and assured Morton of his friendship and his desire to come to an agreement.

The meetings continued up to the Saturday night. On the following Monday the mail steamer was due to sail for Europe, and Morton was anxious to send off on the boat a statement from Jackson affirming that he had made the discovery. On the Sunday Morton called on Jackson at the request of Jackson's lawyer, and they had a long conversation on the subject, at the end of which Jackson said, "Well, I have prepared an article to appear in the *Daily Advertiser* tomorrow morning, which will satisfy, and set the matter for ever at rest."[6] Such a public statement, he explained, would have more effect than if he simply wrote a private letter to Beaumont. Copies of the paper would then be dispatched by the steamer leaving the following morning, Monday, March 1st, and everyone in Europe would soon know the truth about the discovery. Morton asked to see the article, but Jackson excused himself, saying his copy was already with the printers.

Early the following morning Morton rushed out eagerly to get an advance copy of the *Daily Advertiser*. Anxiously he scanned the pages, but not only was there no statement from Jackson that the honour for the discovery rightly belonged to Morton, but, much worse, there was a report of a meeting of the American Academy of Arts and Sciences which was supposed to have taken place, at which, it said, the celebrated Dr C. T.

123

Jackson had read a paper giving details of his great discovery of anaesthesia.

Morton was absolutely dumbfounded. The meeting was actually not due to take place until the following day—March 2nd—and yet here was what purported to be an official account of it appearing in a newspaper printed on March 1st. Quickly Morton read on through the report as Jackson described how he claimed to have made the great discovery—lies from beginning to end, Morton knew. But the article made it seem as if Jackson's paper had in fact been given the official sanction of the whole of the American Academy, and as if they had accepted Jackson as the discoverer, for at the end of the report appeared the names of the most important members of the Academy—Everett, President of Harvard and of the Academy, Warren, and others well known in America and Europe—recommending that Jackson's statement be presented to the Academy. Nowhere was there any mention of Morton's name as discoverer!

Obviously Jackson had tricked them all again. He had got his story printed in the *Daily Advertiser* just as if it had really happened, and had sent copies of the paper off on the mailboat leaving that day for Europe—planning it all carefully so that there was now no chance of Morton or anyone else being able to issue denial before the boat left. Eventually Morton found out what had happened. Jackson had asked to be allowed to read a paper before the Academy on the subject of anaesthesia and had canvassed Everett, Warren, and other influential members of the Academy to let him make a statement. In this he was to have explained his part in the discovery, but far from its being a true account the statement blatantly declared that Jackson was the discoverer. Everett made the position clear later: "I need scarce say that my recommendation to Dr Jackson to address a paper on the subject to the American Academy can in no degree be regarded as giving sanction of this body to his statements."[7]

Having written his paper falsely claiming the discovery, Jackson had then gone round to the editor of the *Daily Advertiser* and offered to let him have an advance copy of his speech. The editor must have thought it extremely kind of Professor Jackson to give him an exclusive report of what he was going to say at the meeting about the discovery the whole town was talking about, and no doubt the idea appealed to him even more when Jackson told him that because of the international interest in this great discovery he would be ordering extra copies of the *Daily Advertiser* to send abroad.

When Bigelow and Gould heard the news they were so incensed by Jackson's trick in suggesting that the Academy had accepted his claim to be the discoverer that they jumped into a carriage and rushed straight off to see Everett to ask him to issue an immediate denial. Later the Trustees of the Massachusetts General, headed by Everett, made a statement publicly reprimanding Jackson for sending to Europe "a statement of his claims to this discovery, when, in fact, it had not been so read; thus communicating it to the world under an official sanction, to which it was not yet entitled. . . . We still find that every part of the statement is utterly irreconcilable with the facts."[8]

But although they condemned his lies, the damage had already been done. Morton could see now that it had all been a trick—and a trick which had succeeded all too well. The March boat had sailed for Europe without the declaration Jackson had promised to give him, and, what is more, without a single word of protest from Morton about Jackson trying to steal his discovery. Even worse, hundreds of copies of the paper had now gone off to the important figures and learned societies in Europe, each carrying a full report of the eminent Dr Jackson describing his discovery of anaesthesia in the presence of, and apparently with the approval of, all the distinguished guests at a meeting of the American Academy. It would be another month before the next mailboat sailed—another month before Morton would have any chance of getting word to Europe. In the meantime Jackson would be firmly entrenched there, all of Europe would have accepted him as the discoverer, and scientists would view with suspicion someone who tried now to establish a claim.

But the amazing thing about Morton was that in spite of all Jackson's deceitful behaviour, in spite of everything that had happened, he still went on working to try to reach a settlement. Whether it was his Christian views which taught him to forgive his enemies, or just his dogged persistence, throughout his life, no matter what happened, nothing could put him off what he had set out to accomplish, and he continued to discuss with Jackson's lawyer the possibility of agreement. All the time the lawyer tried to explain away the ruse and to assure Morton of Jackson's sincere desire for a settlement of the affair. But the weeks went by and still the negotiations dragged on.

Nearly four weeks later, just before the April mailboat was due to sail, Jackson asked Gould to intervene to act as a mediator between them. At Jackson's request Gould called on Jackson's lawyers, and they asked him to be good enough to write his account of the affair so that the exact history of the case could be correctly established and the points of difference between them resolved. The lawyer told Gould that he intended to do the same from his client's point of view, and hoped that between them they could arrive at some account of the affair which would satisfy both the parties concerned. Gould hurriedly drafted his account and handed it to Jackson's lawyer the following day, but once again nothing was forthcoming from Jackson's side, no account from him of his part in the affair, no visit from his lawyer as promised, no reply from them—nothing. (But nevertheless this did not stop Jackson using Gould's hastily drawn-up document against Morton some time later.)

125

Morton became so exasperated with all Jackson's procrastinations that on March 27th, 1847, he wrote to him:

Being desirous that the misunderstanding between us, as to the discovery of the fact that sulphuric ether will produce insensibility to pain, may be speedily and satisfactorily adjusted, I now propose to you to refer the whole matter to some disinterested umpire, before whom all the testimony on both sides, as to the matter in controversy shall be submitted, and whose decision shall be perpetually binding on all parties.

An answer to this proposition, made with an anxious desire for a full settlement of our difficulties is expected today, or early Monday morning.[9]

Jackson replied the following day, March 28th:

Last evening I received your note of yesterday, and now reply that it will be as agreeable to me as it can be to you to avoid any further dispute as to the claims of you and myself, in the discovery of the application of sulphuric ether by inhalation to surgical purposes.

All that I require is impartial justice, and therefore I cheerfully accept your proposition to refer this question to a suitable umpire.[10]

Morton lost no time in trying to reach a settlement, and wrote back immediately the following day, March 29th, 1847:

It only remains for us to select the person or persons to whom the matter in debate shall be referred. If we can agree—I trust we can—upon some one gentleman, I shall be perfectly satisfied. . . . Please inform me what is your choice in the matter and oblige.

Morton felt he was now so near to agreement with Jackson that although Professor Louis Agassiz offered to go to the French Academy on Morton's behalf to tell them the truth about the discovery, rather than risk anything upsetting their negotiations, he refused his offer.

But Morton's hopes were soon to be dashed to the ground once again, for it was only another ruse of Jackson's to delay a settlement, and every person put forward by Morton as an arbitrator was at first considered sympathetically by Jackson, but eventually after some delay rejected as prejudiced or otherwise unsuitable. Name after name was suggested—but to no avail. Time slipped by, and no agreement was reached, for obviously Jackson had no intention at all of coming to any agreement. Now he saw the chance of grasping the entire proceeds of the patent for himself, and all the honour and glory of it, nothing less would satisfy him, whatever the underhand means necessary to secure it. He intended to defer matters until his own name had been sufficiently established in Europe as the sole discoverer of anaesthesia, and he knew well that every week that passed made his treacherous scheme that much easier. Just as at the end of

126

February they had seemed near agreement, so now at the end of March it seemed that an arbitrator was just about to be agreed, but again the mailboat sailed on April 1st, as it had done on March 1st, without a proper statement of Morton's case and without a thorough rebuttal of Jackson's statement to the French Academy of Sciences.

But if Morton appeared to be silent Jackson certainly was not. He lost no time in advancing his cause, and the April mailboat carried letters from him to all his friends in Europe, men like Josiah Whitney, the geologist. Jackson had already written to ask him to press his claim with the various authorities in Berlin; now he wrote further on March 29th, 1847—only a day after he had promised Morton he would accept arbitration—to press Whitney to see all the influential people in Paris to assure them that Jackson was the sole discoverer of anaesthesia and to make certain to tell them that Morton was only acting under his instructions when he administered the ether for the operations. His words now took on a nastier look, for he wanted to discredit Morton and Eddy, not to give a strict scientific statement of his case:

> I wish you would explain to the gentlemen in Paris, Messrs Eddy and Morton's characters, that they may know how much reliance to place in their statements. The whole Eddy family are at war with us, and old Mr Eddy [Caleb] runs round in the streets, and in the grocery stores to tell his falsehoods about me, and to try and run me down.
>
> We have proofs that Morton is a swindler, and that he has tried to bribe his workmen to certify to falsehoods, and that he attempted to bribe one of the printers of *Atlas* to insert an article against me, which had been rejected by the editor. He is accused of swindling with forged letters of credit on persons in St Louis, New Orleans, etc.
>
> I have seen the letter in which he is denounced for these transactions, and shall soon have other proofs of his villainy. I think, therefore, his word is not to be put against that of an honest man.
>
> Do put this matter right in Paris, so far as you can, and oblige.[11]

Jackson's allusion to himself as an honest man would be laughable, if it were not such a sad lie. On the one hand, he appeared in public to be acting reasonably as a professor and a gentleman, while, on the other hand, privately behind Morton's back he was embarking upon a campaign of vilification against poor Morton and anyone else who supported him. Slyly he warned Whitney that these facts about Morton's and Eddy's characters "need not be published, though I think they ought to be made known to any who should appear to be willing to lay their claims before the Academy of Sciences".[12] Telling Whitney that Morton and Eddy were sending testimonials by the next steamer, and that their letters were to be laid before the Academy then, he said: "Let the Academy at all events decline action until informed whether these memorialists are respectable people or not. It is too bad that I should be annoyed by such a man as Morton; or that anybody should pay attention to his absurd claims. . . . He will ultimately be proved an impostor."[13]

These were the depths to which Jackson's envy and malice were now dragging him, for at the same time he offered a bribe to Whitney for carrying out his instructions: "If I am commissioned a United States geologist, I shall write to you to assist me by taking charge of a part of the work"[14]— a tempting promise to a young man of twenty-six then just starting his career as a geologist. In fact, when Whitney returned to America Jackson did give him a job, but Whitney was also to learn to his own cost Jackson's true character.

Morton was dogged all his life by his feelings of inferiority, and too readily accepted the advice of people he considered his superiors, and when towards the end of April Gould and some of the surgeons from the hospital stepped in to try to settle the matter once and for all, they persuaded him to establish his claim first in Boston, where everyone knew the truth. They convinced him that he would be at a severe disadvantage in Europe, and that it would be best for him to come to terms with Jackson in Boston as quickly as possible. If they could manage to agree on a statement which would meet both their points of view it would find immediate acceptance in Europe, and Morton would in this way gain his object much more easily than by trying to fight it out in Europe. Certainly Morton was intimidated by such an august body as the French Academy of Sciences, and felt unequal to the task of convincing them of his claim. He knew also that Jackson was arguing from a very strong position, for Edward Warren wrote to him:

All over Europe, where I have been, this paper [the *Daily Advertiser* of March 1st] has circulated, or its effects are felt, leading men of letters to infer that Dr Jackson is the real and sole discoverer, because he has the sanction of the names of Warren, of Professor Everett, and of the American Academy. . . . Since the report of the meeting of the Massachusetts Medical Society came to hand, Humboldt and the Vienna Medical Society are firmly convinced that Jackson was the discoverer. In Vienna people are already speaking of the administration of ether for anaesthetic purposes as 'jacksonising'.[15]

In face of such opinions it was no wonder that Morton hesitated before finally breaking off negotiations, and when a few days before the May steamer was due to sail Jackson again seemed so conciliatory Gould prevailed upon Morton to hold his hand. Jackson was apparently going round telling everyone that the whole matter was in the course of adjustment, and they all assured Morton that this was so. But the May steamer also sailed without any statement. Finally, it was Jackson himself who brought the negotiations to an abortive end, when he wrote to Morton on May 3rd, 1847, about a pamphlet published by Edward Warren:

128

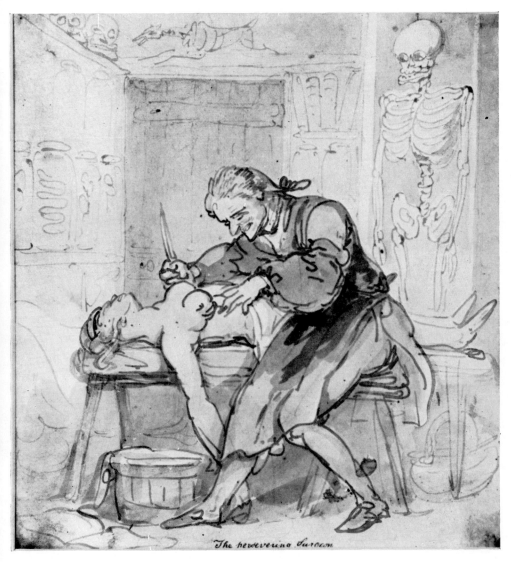

The Persevering Surgeon

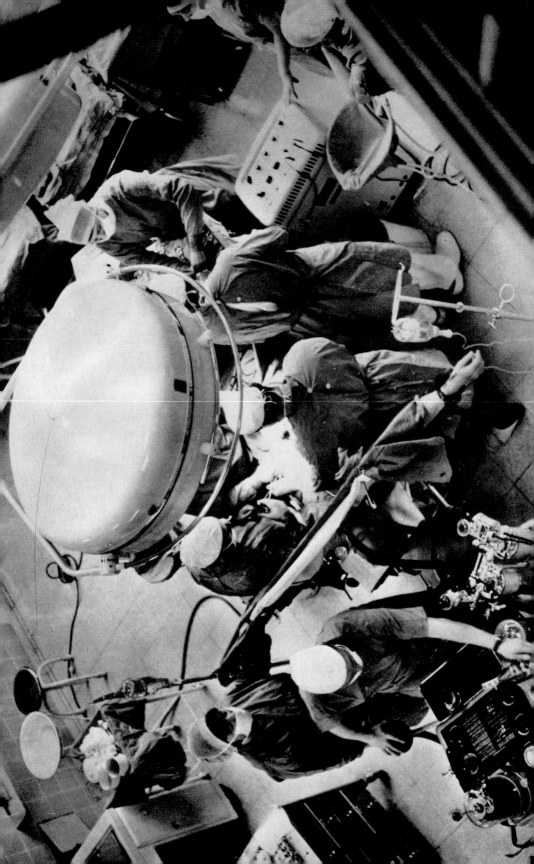

I have lately read a pamphlet entitled "Some Account of Letheon", published, as I am informed, by your consent, and would now inform you that by such procedure, especially by the publication of such a pamphlet, you have absolved me from all obligations to submit our relative claims upon the subject to an arbitration, as was formally agreed upon between us.[16]

So it was to be outright war. Jackson now felt himself to be in such a strong position that he thought he could destroy Morton entirely. Everywhere ugly rumours were circulated against Morton by Jackson or his agents, and Morton's reputation was steadily being undermined. On May 21st, 1847, one of Jackson's students called upon Morton at his office. He informed Morton that Jackson's lawyer wanted to see him on a matter of great importance, one which concerned Morton only and had nothing to do with Jackson. As the messenger insisted that it was a matter of urgency the meeting was finally fixed for four o'clock that afternoon. When Morton got there he found the attorney and the student waiting for him. The lawyer referred to the pamphlet and threatened:

Well, Morton, you know what is in the past; what is to be done? Shall each of you throw all the cudgels he can? It would be much better for you and Dr Jackson to settle than to have the prospects of yourself and your family for ever blasted; for there has been collected from various cities such evidence as must crush and ruin you if it is published. Now, although your conduct may have been the imprudence of youth, as it was before you was of age, still, that will not be taken into account. On the other hand, if you will own the fact that you first got your information relative to the discovery from Dr Jackson and make a statement to that effect, you could stay here, and practise your profession and be a useful man in your business.[17]

So Jackson had resorted to blackmail. Quite what the evidence was supposed to be is hard to say, but Mrs Sarah Hale referred to Morton's early youth, when he had been "duped by designing men" and said that he had had a "silly flirtation in the West that in a youth under age was not certainly an uncommon or unpardonable folly", which "created ill-feeling in the brother of the young lady and in subsequent years lent a shaft to the enemies who have sought to wound Dr Morton since his discovery". Whatever it was, Jackson's lawyer did his best with veiled threats. After inquiring unsuccessfully what their so-called testimony was, Morton lashed out at them: "Am I to understand, gentlemen, that you have sent for me to threaten, and thus to frighten me into your measures? You have the wrong man. You may make the most of your boasted collection of evidence to ruin me and my family. I consider this only shows the weakness of your cause, that you can resort to such contemptible schemes to help it out."[18]

A modern operating theatre

Both the lawyer and the student immediately denied this, and begged Morton to draw up a statement as a basis for further negotiation. Morton replied that there was nothing further to be gained, "as the failure of the former attempt had not resulted from any backwardness on his part to negotiate, but from an evident inclination on Dr Jackson's part to postpone every measure that could bring it to an open and fair judication."[19] The lawyer urged Morton to continue with the negotiations, and said he would arrange for Jackson himself to call upon him. But at last Morton had had enough.

Jackson's version of this meeting was that he ran into Morton at the entrance to the lawyer's office and that Morton had begged him not to publish any of his evidence. But events did not bear out Jackson's statement, for everywhere attempts were made to discredit Morton, and rumours, anonymous articles, and scurrilous statements were circulated about him. In a small place like Boston there was no escape, and his life became utterly miserable. Deeply depressed and disheartened that any human being could behave in this manner, diverted from his proper work Morton attempted to scotch the rumours, but seemed to make no headway. There was to be no end to Jackson's mad and vitriolic hate.

NOTES TO CHAPTER XII

1. Nathan Rice, *Trials of a Public Benefactor*. (Material supplied by Morton himself.)
2–19. *Ibid.*

CHAPTER

XIII

TOWARDS the end of May 1847 it was reported in the New York
Herald and other newspapers that Morton's preparation had been
used for treating the wounded in the Mexican War. Only a month
earlier the Army authorities had said that it was unsuitable for use on the
battlefield, but in spite of this the doctors in General Scott's line had used
it after all. Since no licence fee had been paid to Morton and no permission
granted by him, the Government had in effect unlawfully appropriated
the patent, a patent, what is more, granted by itself. Jackson was one of
the first to realize that if the Government had used the inhalers without
compensating Morton, then anyone could do so, and to all intents and
purposes the patent was null and void. On May 26th, 1847, he sent Dr
Martin Gay round to call upon Morton. Gay was the main champion of
Jackson's cause throughout this affair, and had just published his *Statement of the Claims of Dr Charles T. Jackson to the Discovery*. He came
to Morton's office, again accompanied by a student to act as a witness, and
informed Morton that "the tender conscience of Dr Jackson was troubled
on account of the agreement which he had entered into with Morton, that
he was unwilling to receive the 10 per cent on the profits which he had
bargained for, as he could not but feel that it would burn in his pockets as
so much blood money".[1] With that Gay tore up the contract in Morton's
face.

Morton could not understand it at all, for Jackson had always fought
tooth and claw for as large a share of the patent profits as he could possibly
get. But Morton was soon to see the reason for Jackson's change of heart,
for that same evening the Massachusetts Medical Society was giving its
annual dinner. Jackson had asked to be allowed to make a speech, and
when it came to his turn after dinner he rose to his feet and began,
"Honoured colleagues, as the discoverer of ether anaesthesia . . ." How

131

glibly it rolled off his tongue! He went on to say how he had been swindled into applying for the patent and entering into a co-partnership with Morton, and explained to the distinguished gathering that he had not been told that the unethical purpose of the patent was to make a profit out of the sufferings of humanity. A murmur ran round the room as he dwelt on the iniquities of the attempt to exact a price for easing their patients' pain, and as he talked of the evils of others who had sought to snatch the honour from him and extort their price of silver from the world he was continually applauded. Finally, he ended with a splendid flourish as he stood there and told them how he had destroyed the bond and "voluntarily offered his discovery free to all medical men".[2]

It must have seemed to the assembled company a wonderful act of self-sacrifice and devotion to the cause of medicine, and the doctors seated round the tables warmly welcomed his statement that in future they would be able to use Morton's discovery without having to pay any licence fees. They could see, too, that it was one in the eye for Morton, now widely regarded in Boston as an upstart, and smeared still further by Jackson's campaign of slander and vilification. As in one of their melodramas, whenever Morton's name was mentioned they hissed loudly at the villain, and when Jackson declared his intention to let them have it free he got such an ovation that even the doorkeepers looked in to see the cause of so much noise.

Jackson certainly made the most of the opportunity, and in the hands of every guest was a copy of Gay's pamphlet setting out his case. He had received a great ovation, but during the speech some might have been tempted to ask whether the article in the *Herald* had not forced Jackson's hand, and whether it was not too much of a coincidence that he had only now decided to relinquish his right to profits. For seven months he had held an interest in the patent, and it was odd that he should choose that particular moment to renounce his claim, just when the patent looked like being valueless anyway. They might, too, have paused to consider whether it was really his discovery and patent that he was giving away so freely. But in all that assembly there was only one who had the courage to question Jackson's fine words—Professor Louis Agassiz. Agassiz, well known in Boston for the quickness of his tongue, asked Jackson, "If Dr Morton had killed the first patient to whom he administered the ether by inhalation, would you, who are now so generously renouncing profit from the discovery, also in that case have accepted your share of the blame?"[3] But to this thrust there was no reply, and it was soon lost in the applause.

Jackson's apparently generous action meant not only that in future Morton's discovery could be used without payment by any doctor, but also that it was available for any unskilled or unscrupulous person to use as he liked. Jackson had placed a most dangerous instrument in the hands of all. But why should he care? Now there was no possibility of making any

132

profit Jackson wrote off to Whitney: "I do not care about the money. I have never received a cent, and never expect to receive anything for my discovery; I wish only to receive the honour and to legally fix my claim to posterity."[4] But if it meant nothing to Jackson the effect on Morton was disastrous. Advised that it was useless to try to enforce his patent, he could see there was now no hope of recouping his vast expenses, or of collecting enough funds from the patent to pay for his magazine, or the clinic he had hoped to set up to train operators and to provide information on anaesthesia. All his plans fell to the ground.

As if Jackson had not already done Morton enough harm, only forty-eight hours after he had repudiated the patent at the Medical Society dinner Morton arrived home at his house at West Needham to find a very strange scene. His children were nearly always waiting to greet him, but that night there was no sign of them. Instead it all seemed unnaturally quiet as he hurried up the steps to the veranda. There, striding up and down outside the front door, was a stranger. "Do you not find the family at home, sir?"[5] asked Morton. Curtly the man replied that he had. Puzzled, Morton had started on into the house when his eldest son came running up anxiously to tell him that the rest of the family were all in the nursery. Morton hurried there to find everyone huddled together in terror. Mrs Morton told him that the man had been in the house all day and had acted most strangely. She had met him first driving furiously towards the house as she drove out that morning, and when she returned she had found him in the parlour lounging on the couch with his hat on. It had seemed such rude and extraordinary behaviour to her that when he refused to reveal his business she had become scared and had immediately assumed he must be a madman. She had promptly gathered all the family together, and they had taken refuge in the nursery. She was so frightened that she had even sent for her parents to come over as quickly as possible, and her mother had come to be with them. Who can he be, what can he want, she asked Morton frantically.

Morton went at once to talk to the stranger, but just as he was passing the hall door he was met by a messenger from his office who handed him a letter. The man explained that he knew nothing at all about it, except that a gentleman had called and begged him to deliver the letter immediately. Morton tore it open and read:

DEAR SIR,
I have at this moment learned most singularly of a deep-laid plot to ruin your practice, and to drive you from the State. Were it not that it embraces steps intended to annoy and disturb not only yourself, but your innocent wife and children, and that, through your humane discovery you have saved my life, I should not feel justified in committing this breach of confidence which I do in making this statement.
I can at present do no more than counsel you to guard the impulses of

133

your fiery nature, and trust to Providence that all will end as well as I sincerely believe it will.

One whom you have forgotten, but
who will never cease to remember you.[6]

Morton stood there looking at the letter in his hand. He had no idea who it was from or what it meant. Puzzled, he went outside to challenge the strange man, but on inquiring from him the nature of his business the man only answered insolently: "When that's inquired of by the proper parties I shall be ready to communicate my business."[7]

Morton told him then who he was, and the man immediately apologized profusely, saying he had expected Dr Morton to be a much older man. He had come, he explained to Morton, with an order from the sheriff to take charge of all Morton's possessions, and to stand guard over them until a suit laid against him by a creditor in Boston had been decided. He was, in fact, the bailiff.

Morton was overwhelmed. How could such a shameful thing have happened to him? He questioned the man indignantly—what was this suit, what was this debt, who was he supposed to owe money to? The man did not know—he had merely been instructed to take possession of all Morton's personal property until the debt had been paid. Morton paced up and down the veranda, desperately wondering what to do. He felt sure there must have been some mistake. He knew he was not being pressed for any outstanding debts, and was at a loss to know what had happened or how he was to extricate himself from such an embarrassing situation. Certainly there was nothing to be done at that time of night, and he went to console his wife. He did not want to worry her with what had happened, but assured her that he would soon put the matter right in the morning.

The following day even more puzzling and distressing events occurred. As he was on the way up to his surgery he met one of his patients on the stairs. He greeted him cordially but got the strange reply: "This is a very serious business, doctor; my mother-in-law is in great distress."

"Is there anything I can do for her?" asked Morton.

"Do for her? Why, the very mention of your name would drive her frantic. Her physician has scarcely admitted the members of her own family to see her since her interview with the officer."[8]

At that the patient hurried away, leaving Morton completely bewildered. At the entrance to his surgery he met one of his most valuable patients on her way downstairs. He excused himself for being late, but she answered, "Oh, it is no matter. I shall not want any more attention."[9] And then she too left in a rage. As he went into his office he was met by one of his staff, who told him that there was a lady in the waiting-room in a very agitated state. "I suppose you can guess, doctor, what I'm here for?" she greeted him. "I think they might have been a little more civil with me. Now, doctor, you will not see me go to court, will you?"[10]

134

Morton was absolutely baffled by it all, but for the rest of the day his waiting-room was crowded with patients, some storming in, indignant at what they supposed was his outrageous treatment of them, some pleading with him to stay his hand and not put them to shame in front of all their friends. Others were really rude and vowed never to come near him again.

Morton was completely at a loss for the reason for it all, but eventually, after hearing their various stories, it finally dawned on him what must have happened. Someone had managed to extract from his account books a list of his patients and the amounts they owed him. Writs of attachment had then been served on every one of them, whether they had settled their account or not. Those who had already paid Morton were outraged at the treatment that they supposed they had received at his hands, and the others either hurried to pay their bills and be done with him, or to beg him not to embarrass them by dragging their names through the courts. It was quite unheard of for a professional man to take his patients to court like this, and they were indignant at such shameful treatment. To make matters worse, action had been taken against them in the circuit courts, which allowed attachment of property not only in the state of Massachusetts, but in the other states as well.

Morton tried desperately to explain to his patients that the summonses had been issued without his knowledge, and assured them that he would never have treated patients so dreadfully. But it was useless. No one would believe him. For after all, they asked, who else would want to go to all that trouble and expense to upset his patients and damage his practice? Morton had a very good idea, for he knew now to what lengths Jackson would go to attain his ends. Although Morton protested his innocence, most of his patients refused to believe that he was not responsible for their embarrassment. Convinced that Morton had treated them very badly, they left outraged and went to rival dentists.

Morton was heartbroken. The final indignity came when he arrived at his surgery one morning to find an extra plate on the door. His chief assistant had left him and set up business on his own. The rest of his assistants soon followed. Now not only had his patent been taken from him, but his livelihood too, and when word got around that Morton was liable to be in financial difficulties a mass of creditors immediately descended upon him. Doctors and dentists who had bought licences to use his patent, finding everyone using Morton's discovery freely and their licences valueless, came clamouring for a refund of their money. Agents sent out to arrange the sale of licences pressed for the payment of their expenses, and some even wrote from abroad that they were stranded without sufficient funds and begged Morton to send them their fares home. Doctors and dentists throughout the country rushed to try out the new anaesthesia, and with no equipment handy found a sponge soaked in ether just as effective in unskilled hands as the complicated inhaler

135

Morton had so carefully devised. Manufacturers who had made the inhalers on Morton's orders had thousands left on their hands and hastened to extract what money they could from him. Men for whom Morton had guaranteed loans suddenly without warning received mysterious demands for immediate repayment of their debts, and were themselves forced in turn to press Morton for the money he had so kindly guaranteed for them.

Jackson and his agents lost no time in spreading doubts, and spurred on by them, creditors thronged Morton's doors. Everywhere they foreclosed and pressed their summonses for payment. Morton tried to meet them all as well as he could, but having no money was generally forced to refuse. He worked desperately hard to try to pay off his debts, but with every possible claim for payment pushed to the bitter end he was constantly harassed by a spate of lawsuits for petty debts. Much of his time was wasted appearing in court, and still the claims poured in. He sold everything he could of value, and at one time was even forced to give a bill of sale on his instruments. He begged loans wherever he could, but as fast as he settled one demand he was met by another. Ruin constantly stared him in the face, and his debts enmeshed him. Only the generous action of his friends kept a roof over the heads of his wife and children.

Bowditch, a trustee of the hospital, tried to help him with his affairs, but even he had to report that with all Morton's assistants gone and his patients alienated, however hard he worked he had no hope of paying off all his debts for a very long time to come. During the next five or six months, at his wits' end for money, hounded by his creditors, working day and night to pay off his debts, he had no time to reply to Jackson. The field was open to him to claim the discovery where he liked, and Jackson made full use of his opportunities, circulating memoranda throughout America and Europe claiming the discovery as entirely his and accusing Morton, and Wells too, of being liars and quacks.

The surgeons of the Massachusetts General Hospital were appalled at the turn of events, and the Governors decided to hold an official investigation themselves to make it clear once and for all to whom the honour should be given. They appointed a committee of twelve men, not themselves members of the medical profession and "of the highest consideration in the community". The committee asked the protagonists to appear before them to present their case, but Jackson absolutely refused to do so, denying their right and competence to come to any decision on such a matter. Apart from his first brief account, Jackson had still not published any exact statement of his claims to the discovery, and it was to be some years before he committed himself. When the Chairman asked, "Are we then to conclude that you have no case?" Jackson replied that Gay would speak on his behalf, but when Gay turned up he only repeated what Jackson had said previously, that he had made the discovery back in

136

1842. When H. J. Bigelow asked him why he had not made it public earlier and questioned him explicitly, "Do you expect to be rewarded for letting people suffer during that time?" Gay merely insisted on Jackson's behalf that he had been too busy then to announce his discovery.

Everyone knew that if Jackson had really made such a momentous discovery he would have announced it immediately, at least to his friends. Josiah Whitney was a student boarding with Jackson when the experiments were supposed to have taken place, but he had no recollection of any mention of the subject, or the accident that Jackson said he had suffered with chlorine gas. Whitney, in fact, had actually received a letter from Jackson written on October 15th, 1846, the day before Morton's first great demonstration, but making no mention at all of anything to do with ether or anaesthesia. In it he gave Whitney all the news, talked about a microscope, the Lake Superior copper-mines, the meeting of the Association of American Geologists and Naturalists, and other matters. "My house is at last completed, and so is the big Howard Athenaeum, a brick and stone edifice. . . . What next?" What next indeed! It was a long, newsy letter: "My family are all well, and are now at home. The Plymouth life did them good. I have a fine lot of students. . . ."[11] But not a word anywhere about the wonderful discovery which was to have its decisive test the following day and which he now claimed as entirely his.

The Committee of Inquiry soon dismissed Wells from their consideration, for when Hayward asked him formally if he had ever given sulphuric ether by inhalation so as to render a patient insensible to pain and had performed a surgical operation on him while in that state, Wells had to reply that he had not. Wells had always maintained that nitrous oxide was a better agent, and kept saying that "it is the same in principle if not in name",[12] which was completely untrue. He made it obvious that he did not understand the principles and effects of inhaling ether, for when he had first tried to claim Morton's discovery he had written a letter to *Galignani's Messenger* saying: "The less atmospheric air admitted into the lungs with the gas or vapour, the better—the more satisfactory will be the result of the operation."[13] This proved that Wells knew nothing of the principles, for some air or oxygen must always be admitted or the patient is asphyxiated. Had he carried this into effect during surgical operations he would certainly have killed the patients.

Also, when Wells wrote to Morton about the patent he did not make any claim to the discovery, and Sam Cooley, now a doctor, wrote to Morton: "I know of Dr Wells going to Boston soon after the noise in the papers of the discovery of the effects of ether by you, in 1846, and had a conversation with him on his return, about your discovery. He made no claim to me of the discovery being his, but, on the contrary, expressed regrets that we had not continued our experiments to a successful termination."[14] In fact, Wells's own demonstration at the hospital and a further official one held in the New York Hospital after he had returned from France, proved a failure, and it took nearly twenty years before nitrous-oxide techniques were sufficiently improved for use even in dental practice. Still today there are dangers.

Morton's case on the other hand was already well known to the hospital authorities. He had also now found time to assemble the facts about his discovery and at the end of July 1847 he completed his *Memoir on Sulphuric Ether*. Vetted by Hayward and Bigelow, it was published in Paris in November 1847. In September 1847 his *Remarks on the Proper Mode of Administering Sulphuric Ether by Inhalation* was also published. In his *Memoir* Morton endeavoured, he said, to "state no facts but such as fairly illustrate the history of this demonstration". Metcalf, the druggist, supported his statements about his ether experiments in 1846, saying: "I gave him such information as he could have obtained from any intelligent apothecary, and I also related to him some personal experiences as to its use as a substitute for nitrous oxide, adding the then generally accepted opinion that excessive inhalation (of ether) would produce dangerous if not fatal consequences." Metcalf was able to swear that this conversation took place before July 6th—that is, nearly three months before Morton saw Jackson, because on that date Metcalf sailed for Europe in the s.s. *Joshua Bates*. Morton's contract with Hayden, dated June 30th, also bore out Morton's statements. In his *Memoir* Morton explained also how he had come to take out the patent in the first place:

> In justice to myself, I should say that I took out my patent early, before I realised how extensively useful the discovery would be, and beside the profit motive and remuneration to myself, I was advised that it would be well to restrain so powerful an agent, which might be employed for nefarious purposes. I gave free rights to all charitable institutions, and offered to sell the right to surgeons and physicians for a very small price, such as no one could object to paying, and reasonably to dentists.
>
> I had little doubt that the proper authorities would take it out of private hands, if the public good required it, making the discoverer, who had risked reputation and sacrificed time and money, such a compensation as justice required.
>
> But as the use has now become general and almost necessary, I have long since abandoned the sale of right, and the public use the ether freely.

He closed with the bitter words: "I am the only person in the world to whom this discovery has, so far, been a pecuniary loss."[15]

The surgeons at the hospital, and others connected with the events of the discovery, gave evidence before the Committee of Inquiry that they had never heard of ether anaesthesia until Morton demonstrated it, and that it was not until after the discovery had proved such an enormous suc-

138

cess that anyone else had claimed to have had a part in it. Jackson tried to make out that the committee was biased in Morton's favour, but in fact it was more likely to be the other way round, for Jackson was friendly with them all and the members would be more inclined to favour Jackson, a distinguished professor and scientist, rather than a mere dentist, a nobody like Morton. After a thorough investigation the committee issued its report on January 26th, 1848, with the following conclusions:

1st. Dr Jackson does not appear at any time to have made any discovery in regard to ether which was not in print in Great Britain some years before.

2nd. Dr Morton, in 1846, discovered the facts before unknown, that ether would prevent the pain of surgical operations, and that it might be given in sufficient quantities to effect this purpose without danger to life. He first established these facts by numerous operations on teeth, and afterwards induced the surgeons of the hospital to demonstrate its general applicability and importance in capital operations.

3rd. Dr Jackson appears to have had the belief that a power in ether to prevent pain in dental operations would be discovered. He advised various people to attempt the discovery. But neither they nor he took any measures to that end, and the world remained in entire ignorance of both the power and safety of ether until Dr Morton made his experiments.

4th. The whole agency of Dr Jackson in the matter appears to consist only of his having made certain suggestions which led or aided Dr Morton to make the discovery—a discovery which had for some time been the object of his labours and researches.[16]

Jackson was furious at the report and refused to accept the verdict of what he described as a self-appointed jury. The Chairman of the Committee of Inquiry, Nathaniel Bowditch, was a trustee of the hospital, a son of the famous mathematician and writer on navigation, and a very respected man in Boston, but Jackson went round referring to him as having "caused to be printed an *ex parte* statement in favour of the claims of that quack dentist whom I allowed to use my method of preventing pain in surgical operations, a man of no science, of no knowledge of physiology, nor of medicine, a mere conveyancer of real estate—a man wholly incapable of any scientific examination of this question, and a man of most bitter prejudices against me, personally, exceeding in dogged obstinacy any man I ever knew or have ever heard of."[17] Jackson got his lawyers, the Lord brothers, to issue a pamphlet, *A Defense of Dr Charles T. Jackson's Claims to the Discovery of Etherization*, in which they called Bowditch "a meddlesome fellow", the centre of an "atrocious conspiracy to break down the character of an innocent man and rob him of his rights of discovery, rights dearer to scientific men than money or life itself". How they could talk of Jackson as an "innocent man" when he had tried to rob

Morse, Beaumont, Schönbein, and now Morton of these same precious rights is beyond belief.

In the pamphlet Jackson gave his version of what happened when Morton visited him to ask for a gasbag, supporting it with statements from two of his students, one called Barnes, which were supposed to give an exact account of the conversation that took place. According to this Jackson was supposed to have told Morton exactly how to administer the ether, assuring him it was not harmful, while Morton asked, "Sulphuric ether? What is that? Is it a gas?" Josiah Whitney said Barnes afterwards confessed that his sworn statement had been rewritten by another person, no doubt meaning Jackson or his lawyers.

Jackson also ridiculed Morton's account of his experiments where he said that his dog had leapt ten feet after arousing from ether. To discredit Morton further he picked on fourteen even more minor inaccuracies, and accused him of rigging the evidence, talking disparagingly of "Mr Morton's coterie of witnesses, animated by esprit de corps!"

In spite of all Jackson's lies Morton never became vindictive and merely stuck firmly to the truth of his own statements. He even admitted quite freely his own debt to Jackson:

> I will make a single remark upon the subject of my interview with Dr Jackson. I am ready to acknowledge my indebtedness to men and to books, for all my information on this subject. I have got a little here, and there a little. I learned from Dr Jackson in 1844, the effect of ether directly applied to a sensitive tooth, and proved by experiment, that it would gradually render the nerve insensible. I learned from Dr Jackson, also in 1844, the effect of ether when inhaled by students at college, which was corroborated by Spear's account, and by what I read. I further acknowledge, that I was subsequently indebted to Dr Jackson for valuable information as to the kinds and preparations of ether, and for the recommendation of the highly rectified from Burnetts, as the most safe and efficient. But my obligations to him hath this extent, no further. All that he communicated to me I could have got from other well-informed chemists, or from some books. He did not put me upon the experiments; and when he recommended the highly rectified sulphuric ether, *the effect he anticipated was only that stupefaction which was not unknown, and he did not intimate in any degree a suspicion of that insensibility to pain which was demonstrated, and astonished the scientific world* [Morton italics].[18]

Morton had to call in a lawyer, R. H. Dana junior, to help deal with Jackson's machinations. Dana was a member of one of the most distinguished New England families, a prominent lawyer and a lecturer at Harvard Law School, and famous himself as the author of *Two Years before the Mast*, based on his own experiences in a sailing-ship. Dana gave Morton superb support throughout the whole affair, but was con-

140

stantly bedevilled by Morton having at the beginning given Jackson a share in his patent. "I consider all your present difficulties have arisen from the mistaken advice of Mr Eddy to let in Dr Jackson." Dana edited the documents of the inquiry, promising to be "bound to thoroughness and accuracy" and to "introduce no evidence that I do not believe to be worthy of credit". To counteract Jackson's vicious statements Dana had the report of the trustees of the hospital and Morton's *Memoir* published in the March 1848 number of the magazine *Littell's Living Age*, and arranged for ten thousand copies to be printed for Morton at four cents a copy.

When Jackson heard about it he was furious and persuaded the editor not only to put out a statement of Jackson's own claim, but to suggest that they had been forced into publishing the report in Morton's favour without being aware of the full facts of the case. They also repudiated their original agreement, now demanding twelve cents for each of Morton's ten thousand copies, instead of the four cents previously agreed by them verbally with Dana. Jackson's own lawyers then themselves began proceedings against Morton for payment of the money. Although the affair dragged on for two years, Morton refused to pay their outrageous demand, for he would never give in to what he considered unjust, no matter what the consequences. Eventually he was successful, and the magazine had to settle for the proper four cents a copy, but throughout all this time the case added further to the pressure of his many other worries. Dunned relentlessly by his numerous creditors, maligned by his fellow medical men, hounded by Jackson's malicious schemes, he was pushed almost to breaking-point.

NOTES TO CHAPTER XIII

1. Nathan Rice, *Trials of a Public Benefactor*.
2. *Ibid.*
3–14. *Ibid.* (Morton's own story.)
15. William Morton, *Memoir on Sulphuric Ether*.
16. Nathan Rice, *op. cit.*
17. *Ibid.*
18. William Morton, *op. cit.*

CHAPTER

XIV

MORTON had always hoped that the United States Government would take over his discovery and that they would reward, or at least reimburse, him for the expenses he had incurred in developing it. He had been continually assured by his friends at the hospital and by members of Congress that the Government was certain to do so. He knew that there were many precedents, for Congress had already paid out large sums for inventions—5000 dollars for bullet moulds; 20,000 dollars for an invention for aiming heavy cannon; 76,300 dollars to the heirs of Robert Fulton for improvements in steam navigation; and 25,000 dollars to McCulloch and Booth for an improved method of refining gold bullion. There was even a precedent in the medical field, for William Beaumont had been awarded a gratuity for his work with St Martin. In Europe too discoverers were rewarded, and Jenner had been given £10,000 to compensate him for his practice being "so interrupted in the ordinary exercise of his profession, as to materially abridge its pecuniary advantages".[1] When it was known that this amount hardly covered the expenses he had incurred a further £20,000 was given to him, as well as the £7000 raised in India.

Morton naturally hoped for the same treatment, and almost immediately after the first successful operation had sent Edward Warren to Washington to apply for recognition of his discovery. His application of December 28th, 1846, had been laid before Congress, and Morton had been advised to go himself to Washington to press his claim, but had decided that he could do more good by staying in Boston to promote the successful introduction of anaesthesia. James Dixon, the Member for Connecticut, Wells's home state, had put in a protest on behalf of Wells and had promised to furnish evidence in support, but Wells had already abandoned his work on the subject, and nothing more was heard then. The committee had also

142

received some unfavourable letters on the matter, and Congress was any-way much too busy with the war in Mexico and all the controversies about that to have time to consider Morton's case. There seemed nothing to be gained by staying in Washington, and Edward Warren had come back to Boston.

When Morton heard that the Government had used his discovery for treating the wounded in the Mexican war without paying the licence fees he had been advised on all sides not to try to enforce his patent, but to rely on the Government's remunerating him for it. Still the Government took no action, and the doctors at the hospital decided to approach Congress themselves on Morton's behalf. On November 20th, 1847, Warren, Bigelow, Hayward, and the others submitted a petition to "the Senate and House of Representatives of the United States of America, in Congress assembled":

> The undersigned, physicians and surgeons of the Massachusetts General Hospital, beg leave to represent:
> That, in the year of 1846, a discovery was made . . .
> That a patent for this discovery was taken out . . .
> That the success of this method of preventing pain has been abund-antly and completely established . . .
> The undersigned respectfully pray, that such sums as shall be thought adequate may be paid by the Government of the United States to those persons who shall be found, on investigation, to merit compensation for the benefit conferred on the public by this discovery and on condition of relinquishment by them of any patent right they may hold restricting its use.[2]

When word got round that the surgeons of the hospital had applied to Congress for a reward, all the protagonists and their supporters were alerted. Wells had just returned from Paris expecting to be acclaimed a great discoverer, but instead he found that even in Boston where he was known, Morton had been given the honour. Far from being hailed as America's favourite son, Wells found himself cold-shouldered and remem-bered only as the man who had made such a fool of himself when his demonstration of nitrous oxide had failed. Bitter and disillusioned by his treatment, he tried to marshal support for his claim, but made no head-way. Setting out to discredit Morton, he tried to prove the chloroform just introduced by Simpson was superior to Morton's ether. In fact, chloroform is a more dangerous agent, acting on the heart, not the breathing, as ether does, and so gives less time to revive. Embittered by his own lack of success and the thought of the honour he felt should have been his, Wells spent more and more time experimenting with chloroform.

On his return from Europe Wells had moved to New York and set up business there at 120 Chamber Street, advertising in the New York

Herald of January 7th, 1848, that he was a surgeon-dentist "known as the discoverer of ether and various stimulating gases in annulling pain, now a resident of New York and willing to attend to those who might require his personal services". He tried hard to persuade doctors and dentists to use chloroform, but did not get very far, for they were all quite satisfied with ether and saw no reason to change to something new and largely untried in America. He continued with his experiments with chloroform, using it now on himself. It satisfied his craving for recognition, but soon he became hopelessly addicted, his health undermined and his mind unhinged. Driven by desperation and despair, and maddened by his addiction, he turned more and more to the rosy dreams and release from his painful thoughts that ether and chloroform could give him. Soon he was reduced to a miserable existence where the only people who would have anything to do with him were the lowest and most depraved in the town. Eventually even the prostitutes got fed up with the queer talkative and penniless creature who was always hanging about spoiling their business. Finally even they shunned him. Furious at being rejected, Wells went up to one of them on the evening of January 21st, 1848, and whether he thought he was reacting as a good Puritan, or whether he thought he was avenging another, or what exactly were his motives, is hard to say, but something in the delusions of his seared and tortured mind made him fling vitriol at her face.

In a letter afterwards made public Wells said:

> I had during the week been in the constant practice of inhaling chloroform and on Friday evening last I lost all consciousness before I removed the inhaler from my mouth. On coming out of the stupor I was exhilarated beyond measure, exceeding anything which I have ever experienced, and seeing the phial of acid standing on the mantel, in my delirium I seized it and rushed into the street and threw it at two females. My character, which I have ever prized above everything else, is gone. My dear—dear wife and child, how they will suffer. I cannot proceed. My brain is on fire.[3]

Wells was immediately arrested, and the New York *Evening Post* on January 22nd carried an account of "a diabolical outrage by a man who calls himself John Smith, but whose name is supposed to be Horace Wells, residing in Chamber Street". The man, it said, was "arrested last evening by Officer George Beard and taken to the police on a charge of throwing oil of vitriol at a girl in Broadway". He was held in Tombs Prison for two days. On January 25th the *Evening Post* carried a further report:

> Dr Horace Wells, who was arrested last Friday under circumstances which are fully explained in the following letter, and with apparent truthfulness, committed suicide, on Sunday night last, in his cells at the Tombs. By his side were found, on his bed, an empty phial labelled chloroform, the contents of which he had doubtless taken preparatory

144

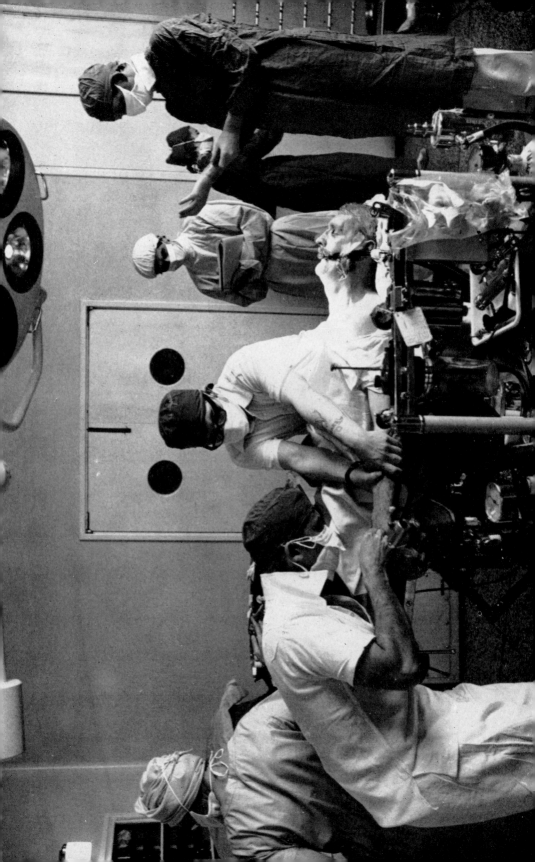

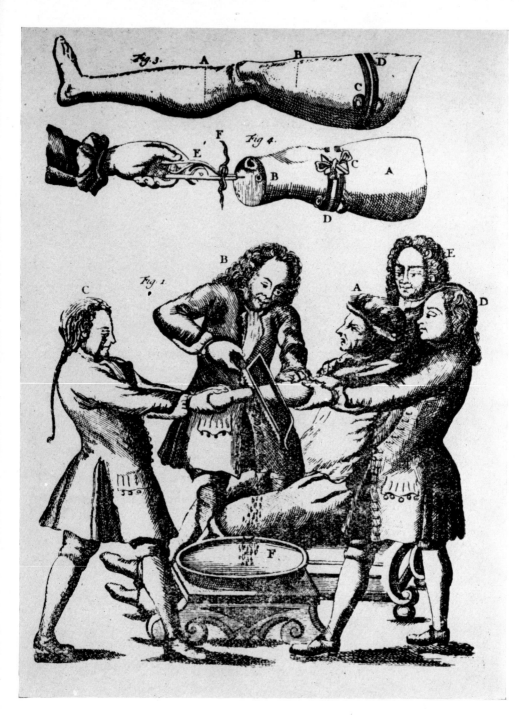

Amputation methods, 1750

to taking his life. A penknife and razor were also on the bed. With the latter he had lacerated the flesh of the left thigh quite to the bone, severing the femoral artery. The verdict of the Coroner's Jury, held yesterday, was that the deceased committed the act during mental aberration. In one corner of his cell were found his watch and the following letters: one to a newspaper explaining the event leading to the disaster; one to a solicitor, and a short note to his wife. The pathetic note to his wife read:

"DEAR WIFE,

"I feel that I am fast becoming a deranged man, or I would desist from this act. I cannot live and keep my reason, and on this account God will forgive the deed. I can say no more.

Farewell.
" 'H' "

Another source quotes one of the letters saying:

Before 12 o'clock this night I am to pay the debt of Nature. Yes, if I were to go free tomorrow I could not live and be called a villain. Oh, my dear mother, brother, and sister, what can I say to you? believing that God, who knoweth all hearts will forgive the dreadful act. Oh, my dear wife and child, whom I leave destitute of means of support—I would still live and work for you, but I cannot, for were I to live on, I should become a maniac. I feel that I am but little better than one already, and now while I am scarcely able to hold my pen I must bid all farewell. May God forgive me.[4]

At his graveside his wife said, "My husband's great gift which he devoted to the service of mankind proved a curse to himself and to his family."

Not long after his death, news was received from France that the Paris Medical Society had elected Wells an honorary member, declaring that to him was due "all the honour of having first discovered and successfully applied the use of vapours of gases whereby surgical operations could be performed without pain".[5] Wells, of course, had done no such thing. He had never used the vapours of gases in surgical operations. He had tried to use nitrous oxide for dental extractions, but even here he had failed.

But it was a tragic ending, and people were shocked by his letters and the manner of his death. Their sympathy for Wells made them turn against Morton even more, and the gossips added to their armoury of abuse the story that Morton had driven Wells to his death. In France a Paris newspaper contended that "while a young, unlucky man who had done so much to free mankind from the curse of pain perished by his own hand with a clouded intellect in some corner of the New World, another, undeserving of the fame he had snatched, was enjoying the credit which properly accrued to the prematurely deceased Wells". Wells had become a martyr, and Morton was responsible.

The pressure of all these events weighed heavily upon Morton. The

K

gossip-mongers, his creditors, rival dentists, Jackson's malicious intrigues, all bore down on him relentlessly until his position became almost unbearable, and his health broke under the strain. Dr Homans, his doctor, declared "from living so much of late in an atmosphere of ether, from the anxiety attending the various trials and experiments connected with the discovery, and from the excitement caused by the controversies which it has occasioned, the health of Dr Morton has become such, that he is unable to attend to his professional duties to any extent".[6] Instead of the thriving business employing many assistants he had before he started work on the discovery, after all those years of hard work he was left destitute, in broken health, and dispirited by his long fight for justice and recognition. Oliver Wendell Holmes wrote on January 30th, 1848: "It is well known that Dr Morton, instead of profiting by his discovery, has suffered in mind, body and estate, in consequence of the time and toil he has consecrated to it."[7]

When his friends at the hospital got to hear of his pitiful state they set about organizing a collection to provide something for him and his family. They planned to raise a thousand dollars among his friends at the hospital, each contributing no more than ten. When Jackson heard about the fund he was furious. He could not bear to think that any sort of help was to be given to Morton, and he put an advertisement into the local newspapers warning "friends of science and humanity" against a "combination of interested persons".[8] He also wrote off to all the people who had already subscribed or were likely to do so, cautioning them strongly against having anything to do with such a project. A similar fund had been started by prominent figures in England to reward Morton for his marvellous discovery. They planned to raise £10,000, as they had for Jenner, but representations were also made to them, and they became so bewildered by the controversy that they abandoned the scheme and returned the money collected to the donors.

In Boston, in spite of all Jackson's efforts, Morton's friends were more successful. Spurred on by the news of his terrible plight they easily reached their target figure of one thousand dollars, and at their meeting on May 12th, 1848, the trustees of the hospital agreed to present the money to Morton, together with a book containing the names of the subscribers and a casket suitably engraved in silver to hold it. A delegation of six of their members was chosen to present it personally to Morton.

All of Boston knew that Morton was in a desperate way, but even the trustees had no real idea of the true extent of the havoc wrought by the burden of his debts, Jackson's malicious attacks, and the constant lawsuits. They were shocked as he stood there before them, worried almost beyond endurance, his heavily lined face looking sick and haggard, and deeply moved at the words: "You will, we are sure, highly value this first testimonial, slight as it is, of the gratitude of your fellow citizens. . . ." The

146

citation went on: "That you may hereafter receive a national reward is the sincere wish of your obedient servants. . . ."[9] As the delegation stepped forward and put the casket into his hands Morton had tears in his eyes as he looked down at the words engraved on the casket: "He has become poor in a cause which made the world his debtor."[10] There could have been no dedication more apt. When Morton thanked them he referred to his pathetic state. Because of "the circumstances in which I have been placed for some time past . . . by my children the testimonial will be appreciated hardly less than by myself".

Morton's fight to get recognition from Congress made no progress, and in spite of his ill-health his friends finally persuaded him to make the journey to Washington to submit his second application to Congress personally. They helped to raise loans to cover his expenses, one of them urging: "I should, if I were in your place, prosecute my claim if I die in the gutter."[11] Morton was so firmly convinced that justice would prevail that he did not need much persuading, and in January 1849 he arrived in Washington, armed with a sheaf of letters of introduction from such well-known figures as H. J. Bigelow, Nathaniel Bowditch, G. P. Putman, and Oliver Wendell Holmes. The day after his petition was presented to Congress it was referred to a select committee, and Bowditch, the Secretary of the Hospital Board, wrote in his letter to the Chairman:

> I regard him as a much-injured man. The system pursued by Dr Jackson and his friends it is difficult to reconcile with a regard to truth, justice and honour. The character of Dr Morton has been attempted to be assailed, his private and confidential letters written many years before, have been procured and exhibited, tales to his disadvantage told with a view to influencing those with whom he had pecuniary dealings, and a deliberate attempt made by Dr Jackson himself to lay before me as chairman of the Hospital Committee, an anonymous newspaper attack on Dr Morton published many years before in a distant State. All this I felt to be an unworthy attempt by Dr Jackson and his friends to procure a decision in his favour, in a mere question of scientific discovery, upon the wholly irrelevant grounds of his opponent's alleged private character.[12]

Everyone at the Massachusetts General Hospital supported him, and a telegram was sent to Washington confirming the findings of the Committee of Inquiry of 1848, "in opposition to the memorial of your opponent". Bigelow sent a letter pointing out that what Jackson claimed to have discovered about the effects of ether in 1842 was only what was already known to the scientific world and set down clearly in print by Pereira. The letter from G. C. Putnam of February 2nd, 1849, declared: "But the discovery, that for which the whole world is indebted, was that the inhalation of ether could be employed with safety—I repeat it, with safety—to annihilate pain. This, the only fact of real practical value, he proved, first by self-experiment, and he was the only man who ever proved it. . . . Let us substantiate the fact that this discovery was made in this country. Let us not decree a tablet on his tombstone, or ask of posterity to pay our debts with a monument."[13]

Morton's own appeal to Congress, dated January 19th, 1849, stated: "Considering the nature of the discovery, the benefit which it confers, and must continue to confer so long as nature lasts, upon humanity; the price at which your petitioner effected it, in the serious injury to his business; the detriment to his health; the entire absence of any remuneration from the privileges under his patent; and that it is of direct benefit to the government, by its use in the army and navy, you should grant him such relief as might seem to you sufficient to restore him at least to that position in which he made known to the world a discovery which enables man to undergo, without the sense of pain, the severest physical trials to which human nature is subject."[14]

The Congressional Committee, composed entirely of physicians, asked Jackson to give evidence before them, but he made various excuses. A mass of testimony was submitted to the Committee, and many people appeared before it to give evidence, one being Nathan Keep, who had asked to be released from his partnership arrangement with Morton almost before it had begun. His letter thanking Morton for his parting present was a very cordial one, and ended that Keep "sincerely wished him a Happy New Year".[15] Now he was conspiring with Jackson to manufacture evidence against Morton and claiming that in an advertisement prepared by Gould on their behalf Morton had fully acknowledged Jackson's part in the discovery. He testified that when the advertisement appeared in the newspaper Jackson's name had been struck out and that he had said to Morton, "Why do you strike out these words? Morton, why do you quarrel with Jackson?" He alleged Morton replied, "I wouldn't if he would behave himself. The credit of the discovery belongs to Dr Jackson, and he shall have the credit of it; I want to make money out of it."[16]

Luckily Morton was immediately able to prove Keep a liar by producing from his files the notes he had made at the time, as well as Gould's original draft for the advertisement written on the back of a letter dated the 9th of July, so that the Committee could see that it was just another of Jackson's attempts to falsify the evidence. Keep also claimed that Morton knew nothing at all about ether anaesthesia and had never allowed enough air to mingle with the ether. On this too Morton proved him wrong, for the specification for his inhaler specially provided for a hole in the side of the vessel through which atmospheric air was admitted. Afterwards the Committee condemned Keep and said his statements "proved to have no foundation whatever in truth", and were the "creation of an excited imagination".[17]

Extraordinary efforts continued to be made to discredit Morton, and

Jackson described Morton to the Committee as "a man of infamous character, and, therefore, wholly unworthy of credit".[18] Scurrilous statements were still being circulated by Jackson's agents, but when Morton's lawyers traced possession of some of these spurious documents to "a certain person" and asked to be allowed to inspect them the person concerned said that the documents were in other hands and no longer under his control. The surgeons of the Massachusetts General Hospital were regaled with unsavoury scandals about Morton, and when one of his employees was asked to call on Jackson to hear some "astonishing things" he was shown letters attacking Morton's character and copies of a western newspaper full of veiled hints. Major Benjamin Poore, a correspondent of the Boston *Atlas*, wrote later: "A common sewer of abuse was poured forth upon Dr Morton who was denounced as having committed every crime, except murder."[19] Nowhere was there left any dirt unsaid, and nothing went unpublished that could possibly discredit him. Disgusting rumours dogged him, and attempts were made to prevent his joining the Freemasons and to bar his entry to all the foremost clubs and highest places. Word was sent to the clergyman of his parish, and even to his own father-in-law.

Jackson's chief aim was to sway opinion against Morton in Congress, and he sent emissaries to the Mayor of Boston to show him evidence and to induce him to use his official position to make representations to Washington to prevent Congress taking any action in the matter, but the Mayor refused. The Chairman of the Committee rebuked Jackson: "It will not do to attack Dr Morton's character, for no man ever came to Washington with better credentials."[20] In their report the Committee mentioned the interviews between Jackson's attorneys and Morton's witnesses and censured Jackson's lawyers for attempts to "entrap him in a mode not usually practised by the legal profession of the United States". They also reported: "A mass of written and printed statements was offered by Dr Jackson, tending to impeach the character of Dr Morton. This your committee rejected, deeming it wholly irrelevant to the subject. . . . Dr Jackson speaks of Dr Morton in terms of great bitterness. He assails his private character, declaring that it is infamous. . . . Much . . . will not be suffered to remain on the files of the Court of Chancery, but will be stricken out for scandal and impertinence."

Morton begged to be allowed to rebut the charges advanced by Jackson, but he was forbidden to by the rules of procedure, and they had to remain on the file and be printed with the proceedings. But the Committee reported: "They deem it just to say, that these charges are not only not supported by, but are utterly inconsistent with the current proofs in this case."

As well as hearing evidence on his behalf the members of the Committee were subjected to a great deal of canvassing from Jackson and his supporters. Jackson himself went round flaunting the letters from Élie de Beaumont, saying that the Committee of the French Academy of Sciences was about to make a declaration in his favour. Jackson had applied for the Cross of the Legion of Honour, and when on January 31st, 1849, the Institute of France awarded it to him he maintained that it was in recognition of his work "as the discoverer of etherization", and sent a telegram to this effect to Congress. The Select Committee had actually already finished its work, but the members were very impressed, and the Chairman of the Committee told Morton that "the despatch was a feather in Dr Jackson's cap".[21] Jackson immediately notified all the newspapers that it had been given to him on the advice of the French Academy of Sciences, who after fully investigating Morton's claim had decided that Jackson was the true discoverer. He then took the matter a stage further by getting newspapers to quote members of the Congressional Committee, saying that they believed Jackson should be credited with the discovery.

But Jackson's lies about the award of the Legion of Honour rebounded, for although he could influence an American decision by such tactics, he dare not risk upsetting such an old-established body as the French Academy of Sciences. He therefore wrote a letter to the *Daily Advertiser* on March 31st, 1849:

> It having been alleged that I have stated that the award of the Cross of the Legion of Honour was made to me by the French Government in consequence of a formal decision, of the Academy of Sciences of France, in favour of my claims to the Ether discovery—I would remark that I have made no such statement, but that I consider the award as due to the entire unanimity of opinion which I have been informed by my correspondents in Paris, and among them M. Élie de Beaumont, a distinguished member of that learned body, prevails among its members as to my right to the discovery.
>
> Under these circumstances I presume the French Government would not deem a formal vote of the Academy necessary—though one may have been passed—before conferring the honour.

Although the main report had already been finished when the telegram was received from Jackson about the Legion of Honour, it so impressed the members of the Committee that some of them asked for a minority report to be added, stating, "It is extremely gratifying to find that our own views concur with the decision which has been pronounced in favour of Dr Jackson, by the most enlightened body of scientific men in the world."[22] The Chairman of the Committee told Morton that had the telegram not been received, "I have no doubt the minority report would never have seen daylight."[23]

But in spite of all Jackson's underhand tricks the Congressional Committee eventually declared Morton to be the true discoverer, and *Report 114* of the proceedings of the 30th of October stated clearly:

Your Committee are satisfied that Dr Morton is entitled to the merit of the discovery. The great thought was of producing insensibility to pain; and the discovery consisted in that thought, and in verifying it practically by experiment. For this the world is indebted to Dr Morton; and even if the same thought, in all its distinctness and extent, arose also in the mind of Dr Jackson, at or prior to that time, yet he did not carry it out by experiment, and thus give it to the world.

Resolved,

That to Dr W. T. G. Morton is due the credit of having made the first practical application of sulphuric ether as an anaesthetic agent, and demonstrated to the world its power to destroy nervous sensibility to such an extent as to enable surgeons to perform all the various surgical operations upon the human body without pain.[24]

The Committee's report should have been a triumph for Morton, but it was already the close of the session. The eyes of the members were fixed on the forthcoming election, and much of the business before Congress was left unfinished. In the circumstances the Committee felt unable to recommend a financial reward at that time, and Morton returned empty-handed, the poorer except for an honorary doctorate of medicine from the University of Washington. Having lost a lot of time and money trying to secure recognition from Congress, Morton came back home to find that his battle in Europe was proving equally abortive. At the beginning he had been fobbed off for many months by Jackson's promises to write to Beaumont and set the whole matter right. Then Jackson had gained a further enormous advantage by getting his paper published in the *Daily Advertiser* and making it appear that his claim had the approval of the American Academy and Edward Warren wrote: "The greatest difficulty I have had to contend with everywhere in regard to your claim had been, and still is, the apparent sanction of the American Academy of Arts and Sciences to Dr Jackson's claims."[25]

Morton could not afford to go to Paris himself, but knew that he must put forward his own claim as strenuously as possible to try to correct the false impressions already established in Europe by Jackson. He was still firmly convinced that the truth would be bound to prevail, and he wrote off to the French Academy to say that detailed proofs would be dispatched immediately. His *Memoir on Sulphuric Ether* had been published in Paris in 1847, and he set to work to get all the many documents prepared, to collect declarations, eyewitness reports, the statements and evidence supporting his claim. Everything was put together in Morton's usual thorough way until he had a really comprehensive statement of his case.

Morton sent it off and waited eagerly for news from Paris, but both Warren and Fisher had left by this time, and he knew no one there who could keep him informed. George Hayward had heard from a friend in Paris that the investigation was progressing well and that Morton should "breathe easy", but ships came and went and still there was no news. Morton expected that all his documents would have been before the Academy during their deliberations, and it came, therefore, as a great shock to him when finally he received a letter from Harnden and Co., written on March 14th, 1849, to say that the boxes of documents he had so laboriously prepared and had printed had been held up at the French customs from May until December 1848. So instead of the French Academy having all the details and sworn statements clearly before them these papers had been sitting there in the customs all that time. Jackson, on the other hand, had been firmly entrenched in Europe for two years, and had been writing busily to all his important European friends by every mail.

Harnden now asked what Morton would like done about the documents. It was an expensive and difficult business, but Morton instructed them to ask their Paris agents to send the papers immediately to Brewster, a young American dentist living in Paris. Brewster had been recommended to Morton as someone who would help all he could, and Morton wrote now to ask him to be good enough to get the pamphlets distributed immediately. Unfortunately Brewster turned out to be a great friend of Wells, the one, in fact, who had taken Wells round the various learned societies there, was in touch with his widow, and was still championing his cause, so he was hardly likely to give Morton his wholehearted support. Morton waited eagerly for news from Paris, but none came. He kept on writing to Brewster to ask what had happened, until at last—nearly three years after the papers had been sent off—he received a letter dated January 1851, saying: "I sent your order expecting to receive a package, but in its place comes five huge boxes. I have not opened them; the day has gone past to circulate these pamphlets. I have no room in my house for them. I have no time to distribute them, and if I did they would not profit anything, the cost of storage will be heavy and useless, therefore, what shall I do with them? Tell me by return steamer. My advice would be to sell them as old paper."[26]

Old paper indeed! Poor Morton, all his hard work had come to nothing. But certainly the day for distributing the papers was long past, for the decision of the French Academy of Sciences and the award of the coveted Montyon Prize was actually made in February 1850. Named after Baron Montyon, who had left a large sum of money to the Academy of Sciences, the prize was awarded to those considered worthy of the title "Benefactor of Mankind". Jackson had at first been accepted as the discoverer, but many of the French doctors had actually used Morton's inhaler and had received instructions from him on administering the ether. Evidence was given that Morton was also recognized in London, but when Beaumont heard the support for Morton he maintained that if the two men had been discovering America it would have been Jackson who was Columbus and

152

Morton the look-out man who shouted "Land ho!" Someone then spoke up on Wells's behalf, but his name was soon dismissed.

The proceedings of the committee were long drawn out, for new evidence was continually being submitted in support of Jackson, while they waited for a detailed rebuttal from Morton. At last, after three years of investigation and dispute, it was decided that some decision really must be made on the award of the Montyon Prize for the year 1848—and an announcement was made in February 1850. Although Jackson had been firmly established with Beaumont and the other members of the French Academy for so long, his case presented impeccably with all the precision of an expert scientist, and in spite of his many personal friends and the lack of a proper support for Morton, the Academy finally came to the conclusion that Jackson and Morton were equally responsible for the discovery:

> Mr Jackson and Mr Morton were both indispensable. Had it not been for the persistency, the far-reaching vision, the courage, not to say the audacity of Mr Morton, Mr Jackson's observations would probably have passed unnoticed and unapplied; but for the observations of Mr Jackson, on the other hand, it is likely that Mr Morton's ideas would never have been crowned with success. The Commission therefore recommends that the Montyon Prize of five thousand francs shall be divided, two thousand five hundred francs being allotted to Mr Jackson for his observations and experiments regarding the anaesthetic effects of the inhalation of ether, and two thousand five hundred francs to Mr Morton for the application of the method to practical surgery.[27]

When Morton heard that the prize had been divided between them he was so outraged at the injustice of it that he refused to accept the prize at all, and for some two years his share of the money remained unclaimed, while Jackson went round saying that the Montyon Prize had been awarded solely to him. Eventually the Secretary of the Academy wrote to Morton begging him to accept the money, for otherwise the prize must lapse. When Morton saw that there was no possibility of the Academy changing its decision he eventually agreed to accept instead a gold medal which the Academy had specially cast for presentation to him. The medal did not quite account for all the two thousand five hundred francs—his share of the prize money—and the remainder was used to pay for a gold frame decorated with a laurel-leaf garland. On one side of the medal was the head of Minerva and on the other the inscription:

Academy of Sciences
Montyon Prize for Medicine and Surgery—1847–1848
William T. G. Morton, 1850

When Jackson heard the news of the presentation of the medal he went round claiming that it was false, and wrote in a later letter to R. H. Bacon:

"That medal affair I think will turn out to be an abominable fraud, and it will break up the last ground for Morton. . . . In order to gull people . . . he has caused by his own order a medal to be made for him by some jeweller or goldsmith of Paris, without the knowledge or consent of the Academy of Sciences."[28] He maintained that the Academy never awarded medals and that he himself had been given the only prize. He quoted M. Jules Marcou, a French Government geologist living at that time near Boston, and insisted, "The Academy has no dies for striking a medal of this kind."[29]

Throughout the world the battle raged as people hastened to show their gratitude for such a marvellous discovery and to shower honours at the feet of the man they thought was their benefactor, some voting for Jackson and some for Morton. In Russia and Sweden they honoured Morton and presented him with the Order of St Vladimir and the Order of Vasa, while in Prussia, Turkey, and Sardinia it was Jackson's turn. Here it was for one, there for the other, and so it went on until the orders were almost evenly divided between them. It was to be a hard and bloody battle, but one which was to continue unbounded for the rest of their lives.

NOTES TO CHAPTER XIV

1. J. Baron, *The Life of E. Jenner*, 1827.
2. Nathan Rice, *Trials of a Public Benefactor*.
3. *New York Herald*, January 1848.
4. *New York Daily Tribune*, January 1848.
5. Letter from Brewster in Paris.
6. Nathan Rice, *op. cit.*
7. *Ibid.*
8. *Ibid.*
9. *Ibid.*
10. *Ibid.*
11. *Ibid.*
12. N. I. Bowditch, *Vindication of Morton*.
13. Nathan Rice, *op. cit.*
14. William Morton, *Appeal to Congress*.
15. Nathan Rice, *op. cit.*
16. *Ibid.*
17. United States Congress, "Report on Ether Discovery", 1849.
18. Nathan Rice, *op. cit.*
19. *Ibid.*
20. *Ibid.*
21. *Ibid.*
22. *Ibid.*
23. *Ibid.*
24. United States Congress, "Report on Ether Discovery".
25. Nathan Rice, *op. cit.*
26. *Ibid.*
27. Académie des Sciences, C. R. 1847, 24.
28. Nathan Rice, *op. cit.*
29. *Ibid.*

CHAPTER

XV

WHILE the battle raged for the honour of the discovery Jackson was busy fighting another, this time for his professional reputation as a geologist. In 1847 he had been appointed an official U.S. Geologist and had engaged Josiah Whitney as one of his assistants. Jackson had been carrying out a survey around Lake Superior when the news came that the hospital inquiry had decided in favour of Morton, and according to his assistants the news had dropped like a bomb among them, Jackson had become even more bad-tempered than usual, and no one could please him. Desperately frustrated in his claim, he took more and more to alcohol. While everyone else was forced to go out into the wilds to survey, Jackson remained in camp writing a stream of letters and pamphlets trying to prove his case against Morton. As Whitney said: "Dr Jackson was averse to hardship, disposed to regard it as a pleasure excursion and lost sight of the great objects for which it was instituted."[1]

Jackson was content to sit about the camp telling anyone who would listen how he had been the first with anaesthesia and the marvellous discoveries of Beaumont, Morse, Morton, Schönbein—he claimed them all—even some of Harvey's work on the circulation of the blood. His assistants constantly chafed under the burden of their conceited chief, and one, S. W. Higgins, previously a topographer to the state of Michigan, said "he could not conceive a more ridiculous attempt of any man thus to depreciate and afterwards to appropriate to himself the labours of others. Instead of being greeted, disgust and dislike met him everywhere."[2]

But it was his misuse of the survey expenses which annoyed his staff most, for he always made sure of paying his own salary in advance, and then if there was no money left at the end of a survey it was his assistants who had to go short. Often the U.S. Treasury drafts went straight into his own bank account, and he drew on them not only for the legitimate expenses of the survey, but for his personal transactions also. As the ether controversy became more bitter, so Jackson became more and more incensed and his behaviour more deranged. S. W. Hill, who ran the Copper Fall Minefield, testified: "One could not well notice the anxiety and interest which he would exhibit . . . without believing him positively insane."[3]

At last his chief assistants, Whitney and Foster, could stand it no longer and handed in their resignations to the Secretary of the Interior with a long list of charges against Jackson. At first Jackson did not seem to be at all worried and readily consented to an investigation. He felt quite confident of his own position, for the members of the preliminary tribunal were all his friends, but in spite of this the tribunal recommended that Jackson be dismissed and that Foster and Whitney should take over the survey in his place. He was again reprimanded: "Dr Jackson will at all times not only studiously refrain from all expressions and remarks calculated to throw suspicion on the motives, or to injure the scientific reputation of Messrs Whitney and Foster, but will sustain and uphold them in all honourable ways."[4]

Jackson promised to send in his resignation on April 12th, 1849, saying that he was about to leave for Europe, but agreements meant nothing to Jackson, and he soon went back on his word and sent off a hasty message to the Secretary of the Interior, saying: "Please do not accept my resignation until you have an explanation from me." On April 17th, only five days after agreeing to resign, he wrote to Whitney and Foster: "I would inform you that I hereby rescind all agreements between you and myself relating to my resignation of my office of U.S. Geologist, and I hereby notify you that I accept your resignations of the appointments that I had conferred upon you as my assistant geologists."[5]

Washington allowed him to withdraw his resignation, and a full public inquiry was held on May 9th, 1849. Jackson tried his usual dodges to gain a decision in his favour, and claimed that his resignation had been forced upon him by "interested parties"; that everybody had been plotting against him; that he had signed the agreement only because he was so exhausted and worried by the vexatious controversy on the ether question and after being advised to do so by friends. But for all his dishonesty Jackson failed again, and on May 16th, 1849, Whitney and Foster received word from the General Land Office that "the labours in the field of Dr Jackson, U.S. Geologist for the Lake Superior District in Michigan, shall be considered closed". The final report also criticized Jackson's behaviour: "In a spirit of bitterness and mortification, he has not scrupled to attack these gentlemen in every point of character, scientific and personal, which stood in the way of his own indication, attacks which were perfectly impotent where the parties were thoroughly known."[6]

Again it had little effect on Jackson, for he immediately began a violent

156

campaign against Whitney, this time to stop him being elected to the American Academy of Arts and Sciences. Jackson was asked to submit his charges in writing, but when it came to the special meeting and the Chairman appealed to him to produce his evidence or withdraw, Jackson just stood there shouting and waving his papers about wildly. Eventually, after an hour of this ridiculous behaviour, the Chairman begged him, "as a gentleman standing in the presence of gentlemen", not to waste their time, but to substantiate his charges. Still he refused. Finally, Whitney's supporters managed to testify that until Jackson's accusations there had never been the slightest suggestion that Whitney was anything but a respectable and honest character whom the Academy would welcome. The members agreed that Jackson's charges were utterly false and brought only out of a spirit of revenge because Whitney and Foster had been made leaders of the geological survey in his place. The result, it was said, should have been "fatal to Jackson's reputation not only as a man of science but as a gentleman".

But they were wrong. The moment Jackson knew that Whitney had left town on a survey he called another meeting. This time a resolution was passed to expel Jackson for his malevolent and dishonest behaviour, but in deference to Jackson's feelings as an old and respected member of the Academy it was not finally pressed. His name and position still counted for something.

It seems incredible that in spite of the failure of all his manoeuvres, in spite of the public condemnation of his behaviour, Jackson still persisted. But his mind was not rational; it was a mad mind, intent on obtaining by any means the power and recognition he insisted was his. Words like truth, honesty, and integrity had no meaning for him, and when in the autumn of 1851 Morton again took up the fight in Washington, Jackson busied himself with his usual style of campaign. Morton had been persuaded to try for the third time to secure an award from the Government when Baron Humboldt wrote asking for "the name of the original administrator of ether for surgical purposes". After all his hard work in Washington it was galling for Morton to receive a letter from the Secretary of State saying: "Your name has been connected with the subject and therefore any information you may see fit to forward hither for the purpose will be transmitted with pleasure for Baron Humboldt's use."[7]

Morton set to work again laboriously preparing a detailed statement about anaesthesia and his claim to be the discoverer. Friends again offered to lend him the money to go to Washington, and he arrived in December 1851 armed with further recommendations from well-known figures in the medical and scientific world. It was an arduous journey, for communications in America were still incredibly bad, with poor roads, wretched coaches, and slow steamers. Washington itself was still not finished and had been referred to as "The Mudhole", or the "City of Streets Without Houses".

The Secretary of State, the great Bostonian Daniel Webster, was very impressed by Morton and invited him to some of the State functions, including a Congressional banquet given in honour of Kossuth, who had led the Hungarians in their unsuccessful bid for independence in 1849. Morton was a guest of honour, and his discovery was talked about with pride by the Congressmen as one of the greatest discoveries ever to come out of America. He was welcomed on all sides, and a Select Committee was set up to consider his petition for a reward.

At the first meeting on December 20th, 1851, Jackson did not appear. After two hours his attorney Hayes finally arrived and said Jackson was unable to come. At the next meeting the attorney was again late, and when he did come asked for a postponement. At the third meeting the attorney submitted that his client was too poor to come to Washington; that he was unwilling to spend his valuable time appearing before them; that even if they arrived at a decision he submitted it had no practical effect upon the world; that posterity was the proper tribunal for adjudication on such a vexed question; that his client, a man of considerable scientific standing in the community, had made a positive assertion saying that he had made the discovery, so the subject should now be dropped. Finally, he claimed it was a decision better made in Europe, and presented evidence that learned societies had recognized his claim, citing the Monyon Prize, the Legion of Honour, and the others.

Jackson took four years to issue his own account in a pamphlet *Etherization of Animals and Man*, but it was fifteen years from the time of Morton's discovery before Jackson presented his case formally in a short book *Manual of Etherisation*. This he very shrewdly dedicated to Élie de Beaumont, by then the Perpetual Secretary of the Imperial Academy of Sciences and a member of the Senate of France. The book opens with a long list of Jackson's honours, and points out that 1846 was a celebrated year in the history of science, for a new planet, Neptune, had been detected, gun-cotton had been discovered, and an agent found to prevent pain. His paranoia had so deepened that of these three marvellous new discoveries Jackson claimed that two had been made by himself. He said he had rejected nitrous oxide because "this gas will not prevent the sensation of pain". But he was quite wrong, for Colton, who had first demonstrated the gas to Wells, did eventually adapt it, performing phenomenal numbers of extractions, and once with two assistants taking out 3000 teeth in twenty-three days. Jackson also made the ridiculous statement that ether and nitrous oxide were "directly opposite in their character", saying that nitrous oxide produced a state of wild excitement while ether was a sedative. His excuse for apparently letting thousands go on suffering was: "It was my intention to revisit Europe and to bring out

158

this discovery in the great hospital of Paris where I felt confident I should be treated with fairness and courtesy; but I was at the time engaged in the geological survey of the State of New Hampshire; and while my report was in the press, was called upon to explore the wilderness of Lake Superior Land District for copper mines, so that I had not one month that could be spared for a voyage to Europe. Hence my procrastination."[8]

The only proof Jackson attempted to give for his whole story was the names of twelve friends whom he was supposed to have told about his discovery. These were all insignificant people like his laboratory students, except for Warren, and he had in fact already declared that he had never heard of this means of preventing pain until it was suggested to him by Morton. Jackson did everything he possibly could to stop Congress from making an award to Morton and got together a petition signed by 144 of the doctors and dentists—not many out of the total of fifteen hundred in the whole state, and most of them merely disgruntled competitors like Keep, or disappointed patent agents who would have to pay Morton if his patent was sustained. Baseless though Jackson's testimony was, Morton soon found himself frantically busy rebutting his evidence. He wrote: "I used to think I knew what it was to be busy, but as I find myself now, I must confess I knew nothing about it. It is trying to keep strained up as I am every moment, and I do hope the day may come when I can sit down quietly, and really have a little rational enjoyment."[9]

His friends rallied round again to bring him support from all over the world. Boott, the London dentist who had been the first to use ether in England, wrote: "Morton is first, and Jackson is nowhere. . . . I still hope Congress will reward him."[10] Simpson wrote to him: "In the monthly *Journal of Medical Science* I have a long article on etherization, indicating your claims over those of Jackson." The doctors of the Massachusetts General Hospital again reported that they had never heard of inhaling ether to prevent pain until it was suggested to them by Morton, but Jackson protested vigorously at the hospital's being consulted, saying that they were biased in Morton's favour and anyway were utterly unqualified to decide upon a matter of such importance. He demanded that the expert scientific opinion of Beaumont and Humboldt should be taken into account. He even announced that if he were given the verdict he would be prepared to forgo any money for himself. Finally, in a desperate bid at the last meeting of the Committee, Jackson's lawyer turned as he was about to leave the room and with some embarrassment remarked, "In pursuance of my instructions, I very reluctantly lay before the Committee these papers pertaining to the character of Morton."[11]

Morton's lawyer, Carlisle, retorted, "Dr Morton is the last man to shun investigation. In my opinion you have done him the greatest favour, that of giving form and definiteness to charges which have been so long set

159

afloat in the community, but which he has heretofore been unable to procure in such a form as to admit of a refutation."[12]

It was again a victory for Morton, for the Committee in their report of April 1852 stated that it was only after he had successfully established ether as safe that other people had laid claim to the discovery. "Great Britain, France and all other enlightened nations," they reported, "have, from time immemorial, rewarded munificently such services to humanity. The British Parliament, by two successive statutes, bestowed upon Jenner the sums of ten thousand and twenty thousand pounds for the discovery of vaccination. The world has as yet produced but one great improvement in the healing art deserving to be ranked with that of Jenner."[13] They therefore recommended that as the discovery had been used freely by the Army and Navy an award should be made to Morton on condition that he surrendered his patent to the Government, and a Bill was prepared for the payment of 100,000 dollars to him. The news was received at the same time as another piece about Jackson. An editorial appeared in the Boston *Daily Mail*:

> "Washington, March 15th. The Committee in the House have decided upon awarding $100,000 to Dr Morton for his discovery of ether. Dr Morton has caused the arrest of his competitor, Dr Jackson, for libel."
>
> The statement is false in many respects. Dr Jackson has not been arrested for libel, although it is true that a majority of the Committee have decided to recommend an award of $100,000 to the discoverer of anaesthetic properties of sulphuric ether. It is rumoured that the Committee were *Mortonised*. A minority report of the Committee to whom the matter was referred, will undoubtedly expose one of the most stupendous attempts that has ever been made to defraud the United States government, by false evidence, the exhibition of a fraudulent medal (from the French Academy of Sciences) and . . . Morton has no more claim to this discovery than the Fiji mermaid; his entire merits in the premises are precisely the same as those of a thief who enters a person's house, and finding some valuable article, attempts to appropriate it to his own use and behoof on the ground of discovery. The attempt to pull the wool over the eyes of members of Congress is in perfect character with the unblushing impudence of the individual.

It was not necessary to go far to find the author, and when Bowditch took it to the newspaper office to ask indignantly on whose authority the editor had published it he was answered in two words: "Dr Jackson's." When his disgraceful conduct was challenged he retreated as usual and wrote to the *Baltimore Sun*: "I have not been arrested in Washington, although a suit has been commenced against me, but upon what grounds of action I am wholly unable to say. I am exceedingly desirous that all the

160

Modern operation for removal of the larynx

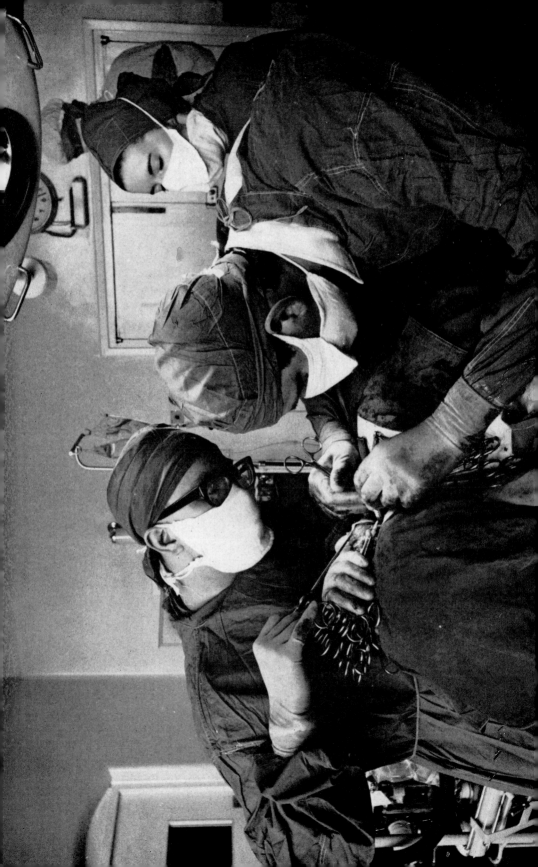

9

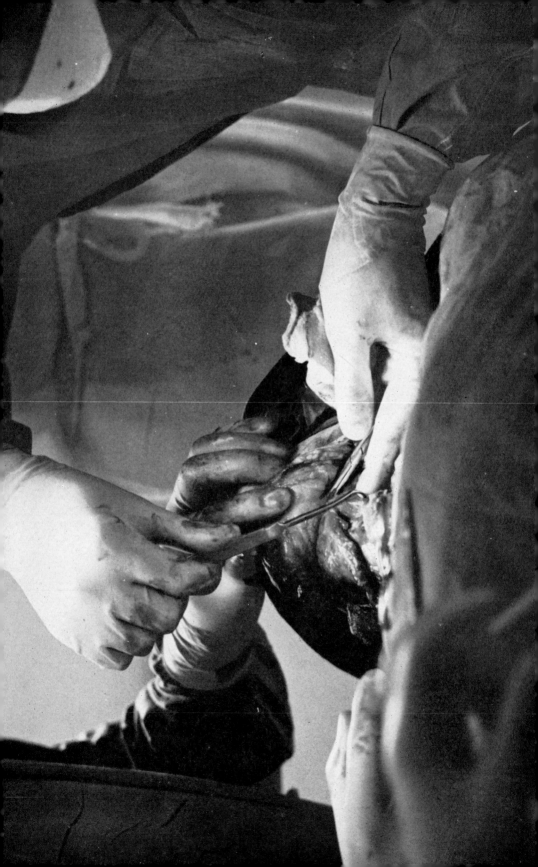

matters in controversy between Mr Morton and myself should be the subject of judicial investigation."

Morton had neither the time nor the inclination to prosecute Jackson, but hoped that it would make him stop his scurrilous statements. Instead he waited happily for the fulfilment of all his hopes and dreams of the last few years—the award to him of the 100,000 dollars. Now deep in debt—with loans extended to him by all his friends—and weak in health, he was in great need of money to release him from some of his burdens. Excited at the thought of the life which was to begin afresh for him and his family, he began to make plans again for setting up his clinic. The Bill was introduced on August 28th, 1852, warmly recommended by the Select Committee, supported by both the Committees for Military and Naval Affairs, and so expected to pass through easily. Congress met in what is now the Supreme Court building, and the Bill was moved by Senator Borland of Arkansas. Making a passionate speech on its behalf, he claimed that Morton's discovery was one of the most valuable remedial agents that the world had ever known, which saved thousands upon thousands of dollars every year: "We are making use of his property to our great benefit, and he is receiving no compensation whatever for it. . . . When was there ever before us a more meritorious case? . . . How can we, then, in justice to ourselves, in common justice to the individual who has furnished us this . . . invaluable remedy, refuse to pay him for it?"[14]

The Senators were very impressed as they sat there listening thinking of their own relatives who had suffered the torments of operations and been saved from their agonies by Morton's discovery. They were all deeply grateful and vied with one another to rise and praise him. Then Truman Smith, the Senator for Connecticut, got slowly to his feet. The members sat silent and horrified as his voice rang out through the chamber: "I denounce this attempt to filch money from the Treasury, as an outrage upon the rights of others, and a most abominable imposition on this government. . . . I believe, that this Morton is a rank impostor—that there is no justice or truth in his pretended claim. I demand," he thundered, "in the name of justice and right, to have an opportunity to come before the Senate, and tell the story of the wrongs of the poor widow and defenceless children of Dr Horace Wells; wrongs which they have suffered at the hands of this man, Morton, who has attempted to rob their husband and father who has descended into the grave, of a discovery, which is one of the most extraordinary made in modern times."

His voice quivered with emotion and indignation: "Will the Senate act . . . in this *ex parte* manner? . . . Why does not this patentee assert his rights? If," he said, sneering contemptuously, "he has got any rights under his patent, why does he not sue somebody for their violation?"[15]

Morton could hardly believe it. Throughout the whole affair he had been constantly criticized for having patented his discovery; now here in

L   161

Operations lasting hours and needing great precision and care are possible today with modern methods

Congress it was being held against him that he had made no move to assert his rights.

Immediately Smith had finished Senators leapt to their feet in defence of Morton and his discovery. Senator Shield attacked Smith and said that if this remedial agent had been known when Smith said, it was unpardonable that it was not used for the American Army in the war, and criminal for Wells to have withheld his information when it would have saved thousands of lives. Senator Douglas joined in to say that Morton had risked his own life by experimenting upon himself, and that he alone had introduced it and taken the whole responsibility of using it "until its entire success had been established".

The Senators sat amazed at the way the debate was going when Senator Badger of North Carolina got swiftly to his feet. "I know not, Mr President," he said, "what private griefs the honourable Senator from Connecticut has; but, certainly something or other seems to have stimulated him into a very undue excitement on this occasion, one not usual upon questions of this kind and one which certainly that Senator is not in the habit of exhibiting in the Senate!" A murmur ran round the House. "The honourable Senator demands an opportunity of making out a case—for whom? For clients of his?"[16]

The cat was then out of the bag, and the Senators roared with laughter as Smith jumped to his feet to answer, but instead slumped back into his seat looking very uncomfortable. Knowing Truman Smith, they might have been a little more suspicious of his apparent concern for Wells's poor widow and children. In fact, Smith was not only the member for Connecticut—Wells's home state—but was also acting as attorney to Wells's heirs. He had offered to lay their petition before Congress and personally to present their claim to the 100,000 dollars, with no doubt a fee for himself into the bargain. What was clear was that he did not know what he was talking about, for he made the same mistake as his client Wells when during the debate he confused ether with 'laughing gas'.

Disgusted at the way the debate was going, Senator Walker stood up to say that there had now been two reports from the Massachusetts General Hospital, two Select Committees of the House of Representatives, both the Military and Naval Affairs Committees—all had supported Morton; a casket had been presented, medals, the Montyon Prize, honours of every sort had been showered upon him, what else, he asked them, what else did members of Congress need in order to convince themselves that Morton was the true discoverer of ether anaesthesia? What else must he do to gain his just reward?

A further interruption came from Senator Hale: "I desire to state a fact which has come to my knowledge since this discussion commenced. I do not know whether it will have any influence upon the votes of Senators tonight; but there is a gentleman in this chamber now who has informed

162

me, and he is ready to pledge his honour and reputation to it, that neither Dr Morton, nor Dr Jackson, nor Dr Wells, has anything to do with the original discovery of this principle; that it was discovered and applied to practice in the City of New York by a young physician who is now in his grave; that if there is any credit belonging to it at all, it belongs to him, and if there is any meritorious reward due to anybody, it is to his orphan sister. The gentleman is ready to pledge his honour and reputation that if the subject is postponed until December he can by irrefutable proof establish the fact to the satisfaction of any tribunal."[17]

Widows and orphans, voices from the grave, they all spoke against Morton. No inkling was ever given as to the mysterious stranger, no proof given; it seemed all part of a massive conspiracy against poor Morton. The debate was drawing to a close. Senator Mallory claimed that the demand for reward had come "from thousands of our fellow-citizens, in every walk of life, whom gratitude has made eloquent. It comes from the lowly couch of the poorhouse patient, and from the aristocratic mansion of the millionaire. . . . Men of undoubted courage . . . shrunk with undefined terror from the prospect which the cold-blooded torture of the surgeon's knife holds before their eyes. . . . The knife has lost its terrors. . . ."[18] He went on: "We cannot pay Dr Morton. His services are beyond price; but we can place his future life beyond the reach of poverty, and in this manner do justice to ourselves. . . . Fulton's merits were disregarded, and he was suffered to die owing more dollars than would have covered him in his grave."[19]

But it was no use, there was no hope of justice being done, and when Senator Truman Smith said, "I pledge whatever reputation I have, that if the Senate will allow me, at the next session of Congress, an opportunity to be heard on this subject, I will make out a case for the family of Dr Horace Wells, deceased,"[20] his intervention was enough to decide Congress against recompensing Morton. The Bill was defeated, with seventeen members voting for it, twenty-eight voting against, with fifteen members absent. The award was again postponed; yet another Senatorial Subcommittee was to be set up to examine the evidence and the claim on behalf of Wells.

Hopelessly dispirited, tired out by his long fight, sick in body and mind, Morton left for home. There he succumbed again to illness from which but for careful nursing he would have died. He wrote to a friend:

I have become a perfect sensitive plant. I am chilled by the slightest changes of weather; a little extra fatigue brings on a spasmodic action, from which I can obtain relief only by warm drinks and external applications. My nervous system seems so completely shattered that a trifling surprise or a sudden noise sends a shock all over me. I am so restless that I cannot lie or sit long in any position, by day or night. Then convulsive pains seize me suddenly, without any premonitory warning or apparent cause, and my limbs are instantly drawn up by the intensity of the

163

cramps, which wrack me so that I cannot prevent screaming until I fall exhausted. . . . After the subsidence of one of these attacks, my limbs tremble, and I feel dizzy, weak, and despondingly sick. The disorder has not diminished for the last four years, but seems rather to increase in the frequency and severity of the attacks.[21]

NOTES TO CHAPTER XV

1. *Full Exposure of C. T. Jackson's Conduct, leading to his discharge from Government service.*
2. *Ibid.*
3. *Ibid.*
4. *Ibid.*
5. *Ibid.*
6. *Ibid.*
7. Nathan Rice, *Trials of a Public Benefactor.*
8. Charles T. Jackson, *A Manual of Etherization.*
9. Nathan Rice, *op. cit.*
10. *Ibid.*
11. *Ibid.*
12. *Ibid.*
13. United States Congress, "Report on Ether Discovery", 1852.
14. United States Congress, Report on Proceedings.
15. *Ibid.*
16. *Ibid.*
17. *Ibid.*
18. *Ibid.*
19. *Ibid.*
20. *Ibid.*
21. Nathan Rice, *op. cit.*

CHAPTER

XVI

WEAK and ill though he was, Morton insisted upon dragging himself to Hartford, where Wells had practised, to collect evidence to refute the claim by Wells's heirs. He arranged also for two lawyers to take sworn evidence before a United States Commissioner, and notices were served on Mrs Wells and others to appear before them. A great friend of Wells, a Dr Marcy, testified that Wells had known about ether because he had used it himself to perform an operation on a patient in 1845. Morton immediately publicly offered a handsome reward if this patient would come forward, or anyone who was able to substantiate the story, but of course no one was found to take up his offer. It seemed incredible that the claim for Wells was ever taken seriously, but again hiding behind the skirts of Wells's widow was Jackson, offering to help her put forward a claim to the money.

A new Congressional Committee had now been appointed, and Morton's friends urged him to go to Washington to petition Congress for the fourth time. "Stick to your aim, the mongrel's hold will slip", wrote Oliver Wendell Holmes. Despite his promise to furnish evidence nothing had been heard from Smith or Jackson, and Morton requested them to present their testimony. Still they delayed, until on January 3rd, 1853, when General Cass came to address Congress and everyone was eagerly waiting for him to speak, Smith got up to propose a resolution asking that the ether controversy be referred to the Committee on Patents. By choosing such an inconvenient moment he hoped to have the matter further delayed, and, indeed, General Cass became so impatient at being kept waiting that he did ask for Smith's petition to be postponed. The following day it was suggested it might go again to the Military Affairs Committee, but Senator Shields protested that it had already been discussed to death by them. Eventually one further special Select Committee was set up, this time under Senator Walker.

As the members of the new Committee had no time to read all the vast volume of evidence laid before previous Committees, Morton had a thousand pages of testimony hurriedly printed at his own personal expense and given to them on January 21st, 1853, together with a draft of a Bill. Jackson and Truman Smith retaliated by circulating their case, *An Examination of the Question of Anaesthesia,* in which Morton was heartily abused, while Wells—and Jackson for his help in the affair—were praised beyond belief. Smith maintained that he was interested in nothing but the truth and wanted only justice for the dead Wells, but just the same he and Jackson used all their old tricks of delay and slander. As Morton said in his petition to Congress of January 21st, 1853:

"It is now more than six years since the world received, at my hands, what I may not scruple to call one of the greatest of physical blessings. Whatever attempts may be made to throw doubt upon other points in the case, no one has been reckless enough to deny that I alone have been, in fact, the humble instrument through whom a beneficent Providence has conferred this boon upon mankind. . . .

"To me alone, of all the world, this result has been fraught with suffering instead of comfort. Of pecuniary sacrifices I will not speak, but surely it was not to have been anticipated that this discovery should have made me the target for the most malicious and envenomed assaults. These are the wounds which are sharper than those of the surgeon's knife, and which,

—Not poppy, nor mandragora,
Nor all the drowsy syrups of the world,

can make us feel less keenly. These have been my portion. I trust that the reward is at hand. I look to you for justice: nothing more," and, he said, "nothing less."[1]

It was a pathetic plea, but again the Committee had to condemn Jackson's attempts to blacken Morton's character: "Arguments such as these, which have no foundation save in the positive imagination of the coiner, show the real weakness of the cause they are intended to sustain, backed by gross libels and defamatory charges."[2] This time, however, the Committee was bewildered by the great weight of evidence and suggested that only a judicial inquiry could recommend an award.

When the matter came up again Senator Walker said: "I have seen a member of my family . . . suffering under the surgeon's knife, lying in a calm and peaceful sleep, and yet undergoing one of the most torturing surgical operations in the world. I felt at that day, rising in my heart, the feeling that if God should ever give me the opportunity of manifesting my gratitude to the person who made this great discovery I should do so. The opportunity is now offered."[3]

When someone asked why Morton did not enforce his patent Senator

166

Borland replied: "You cannot go into the sick chamber and arrest the surgeon in the performance of his professional duty, and deprive a patient, who is on the verge of the grave, of a benefit from the application of a remedy, because it may infringe the right of a patentee."[4]

The Committee report was passed in the Senate, but failed in the House of Representatives. There, when a friend of Jackson's moved to let the court divide the award between the various contestants, everyone in the chamber was immediately on their feet to shout, "A bargain! A bargain!" Certainly it was a most unfortunate time, for after 1850 the two Houses were so completely occupied with discussing slavery that they hardly ever found time to agree on anything. So the thirty-second Congress adjourned and Morton went home, again empty-handed. But not for long. When the Thirty-third Congress opened all his friends in Congress assured him that this time it was absolutely certain to go through unopposed, but this time when he called the attention of the Senate to the Bill on April 19th, 1854, he found himself faced by yet another claimant, Crawford Long of Georgia.

Long had experimented with ether, but been too scared to go on using it. He had no idea of the importance and had not bothered even to record his experiments. In fact, he had apparently forgotten all about them until he read in the medical journals of Morton's great success. At last, in 1849, seven years after his experiments, and three years after Morton had successfully introduced anaesthesia into standard medical practice, Long had written off to the Georgia Medical Society: "I know that I delay the publication too long to receive any honour from the priority of the discovery, but having by persuasion of my friends presented my claim before the profession, I prefer that its correctness be fully investigated before the Medical Society." Long was honest about his failure and said: "Should the society say that the claim, though well founded, is forfeited by not being presented earlier, I will cheerfully respond, 'So mote it be.'"[5]

But this was enough for Jackson. When he saw that Wells's claim was likely to fail he set off south to track down Long and to persuade him to join in the fight against Morton. Long had moved to Athens, Georgia, where he had built up a very successful practice and owned a plantation and slaves and a drug-store. He was still something of a dandy and lived, like any Southern gentleman, a life of some ease and luxury, playing an occasional game of croquet, with whist in the evenings. He had done little to claim the discovery, and was very surprised when Jackson came to see him on March 8th, 1854, to ask about the two operations he had performed with ether. Long was most flattered to think that such an eminent scientist should take an interest in his modest practice, and when Jackson seemed so insistent that he should be given the credit for this world-shattering discovery Long was only too happy to talk to him and to search through his papers and files. Laboriously he went right back through the years until he came to an old and faded receipted account for the year 1842 which proved that Venables had paid him two dollars for removing the tumour.

Jackson urged Long to put in a claim to Congress, assuring him that he was entitled to the 100,000 dollars. He even helped to arrange for statements to be taken from witnesses. But what Jackson did not mention was that he was still continuing his claim to have preceded Long with his own experiments that he said he had done in 1838. But if he could only manage to get Long's priority recognized Morton would be finished, and he would then be able to proceed with his own claim.

So, as Morton's friends sat in Congress waiting for the matter to go through unopposed, Senator Dawson rose to claim the honour—this time for Long, a citizen of Georgia and a Southerner. It made a great impression, but hardly had the members recovered from this surprise when another claimant appeared on the scene, a Dr Wilhite, who had apparently anaesthetized a Negro boy with ether. And then another claim was put forward, and another, and the battle began to rage, North against South, one claimant against the other, each state with its own favourite. Morton, Wells, Jackson, Long, Wilhite, a Dr Justine of New York, a Dr Dickinson, a Dr Marcy—all claimed the discovery, all determined to get the 100,000 dollars.

Soon they were joined by others, even from abroad. A Dr Robert Collyer claimed he experimented in London, and again in New Orleans, but admitted that he had never used ether at all. "It is true that I administered neither laughing gas nor ether, but alcoholic vapour. But surely this makes no difference to the question of priority?"[6] he said! A worthier case was made out for Hickman, who had first demonstrated the effects of laughing gas before the learned societies of London and Paris. Claims poured in, and petitions were even received from the mesmerists. There was little in any of them, but it cost Morton a great deal of time and money to repudiate them.

Morton was weary of the struggle. As he said in his plea to Congress: "You will perceive, Mr Chairman and gentlemen, that the strategy of my opponents is directed to wearing out my life and exhausting my means, in order that they may be in at the death. . . ."[7] So much time had passed, so many fine words had been spoken, and Morton's fight for recognition was still not done. Passed once more in the Senate by twenty-four votes to thirteen, it was finally sent to the House of Representatives, only to be called up quite suddenly and unexpectedly on a day which was supposed to be confined to private Bills. A vote not to discuss the matter was carried by eighty votes to forty-six; a further vote was then hurriedly passed to reconsider the vote, and to lay the motion to reconsider it also upon the table, a procedural move which was used to stop the discussion of slavery, and effectively stopped the Bill being brought before Congress ever again.

168

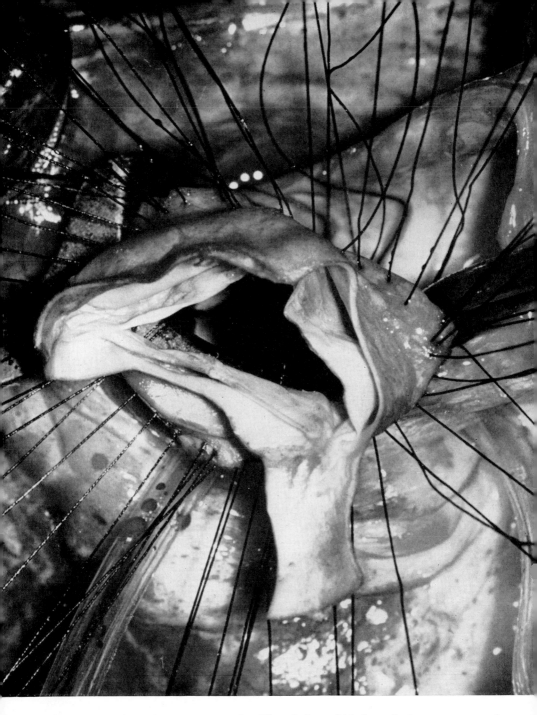

A heart operation today to renew a valve. The stitches, of black synthetic cotton, are made individually rather than by continuous thread

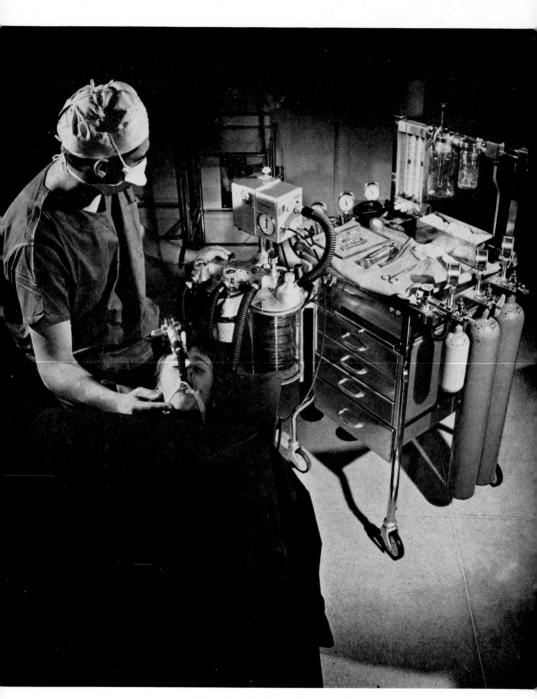

A modern machine for administering anaesthetics

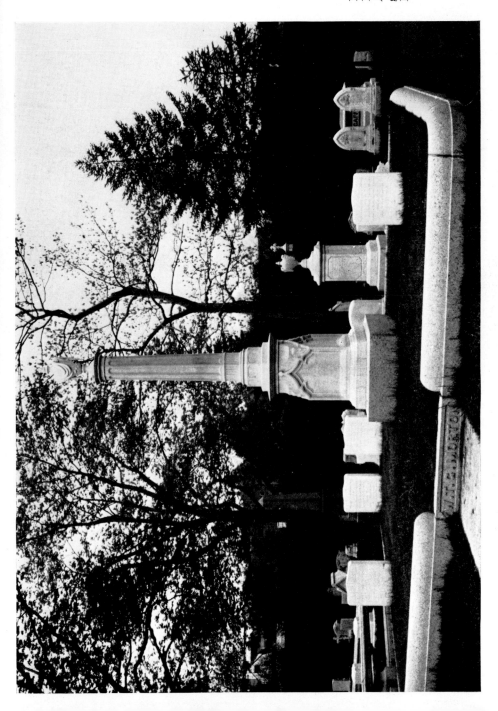

Monument erected over Morton's grave in Mount Auburn Cemetery by the grateful citizens of Boston

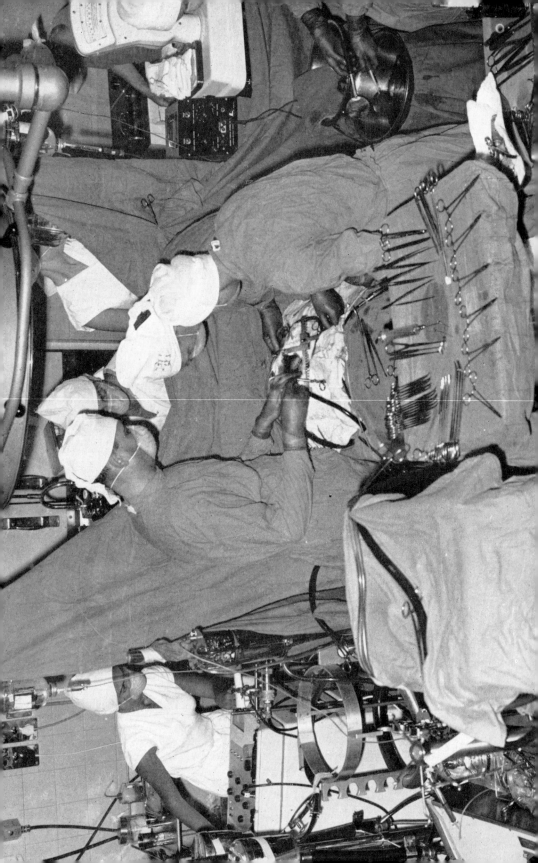

It was finished. After nearly eight long years of bitter battle it was all over, and Morton returned to his home the poorer in time, money, health, and spirit. On April 24th, 1854, Mrs Morton wrote to a friend in Washington:

> I have offered to write to you today for the Doctor for indeed he feels too sick at heart to write himself. You, of course, have seen the papers that his bill was lost in the House; I do not know that his hopes for the future are lost, but his feeling of disappointment now is terrible. He says he feels he has done everything he could do, and yet this misfortune has followed him. . . . We had much reason to hope for success, it passed the Senate with but little trouble. . . . Colonel Bissell came in too late to do anything effectually about it, and . . . the friends of the bill could not obtain the floor to do it justice. . . . It is said to be a matter unknown for the Speaker to go to the business on the Speaker's desk without a motion from a member. . . .
>
> The Doctor's health is so injured by such anxiety and excitement that I feel in no matter reconciled. . . . Do not think he is disheartened or entirely discouraged, for he would not admit that.[8]

Although discouraged Morton returned to his home, this time determined to build a new life for himself and his family, to devote more time to the world he came from, to farming and agriculture—a world of peace and harmony. Some years before, on the forty acres of land he had bought at West Needham, he had built a cottage for his family and called it Etherton in honour of his great discovery. Now, with money from his friends and with his usual hard work and dogged determination, he set out to make it into a model farm. In between visits to Washington he had already begun to make careful observations on different breeds, the fattening of animals, the various fertilizers, drainage, and the essential elements for the vitality and growth of crops—all "illuminated by the light of science".

Mrs Sarah Hale wrote: "Dr Morton has relinquished his profession and now passes his summers entirely at his country residence and his winters in Washington where he hopes to gain from Congress some reward for his great discovery of etherisation. . . . Not a word is heard of ether or chloroform at Etherton. . . . It was all pigs and cows, poultry and farming." It had a steam-engine for cutting and grinding the fodder, a furnace for steaming the potatoes, hydraulic machinery for pumping up water from the stream, "everything," says Mrs Hale, "managed with scientific skill and order". He had many unusual breeds of animals and birds, including a pair of Chinese geese, a present from Daniel Webster. "But," goes on Mrs Hale in her over-romantic way, "within the barn was a lovelier spectacle. From the centre beam hung a large rope, its lower end passing through a circular board . . . thus forming four compartments, with the centre rope for a resting-place. In these snug spaces were seated the four beautiful children, like birds in a nest, swinging every way in turn as the little feet that first touched the floor gave impulse.

169

Professor Christiaan Barnard's operating theatre at the Groote Schuur Hospital, Cape Town

"It was a lovely picture of childhood made happy by parental care for the amusement of infancy. The father's genius had designed that swing for pleasure, as it had discovered the elixir for pain, by taking thought for others."[9]

But it was not a happy time just then in Boston, for the North was shocked by what was happening to the Southern slaves. When on June 2nd, 1854, a runaway slave was forcibly transported from the free soil of Massachusetts to be sent back in chains to slavery and his Southern master, the stores of Boston were all closed, vast crowds gathered on the sidewalks, and the main streets were draped in mourning black with a huge coffin suspended over State Street.

Still Morton did not give up his great cause entirely and on June 15th, 1854, he addressed a petition, this time to the Secretary of State and to the President to try to satisfy the members of Congress who thought that he should enforce his patent:

> The undersigned . . . relying upon the justice and magnanimity first of his own government . . . has not hitherto exercised his legal rights by suit at law for damages, or injunctions to prevent the use of a discovery which has happily proved so beneficent to humanity. Nor would he now take any step by way of departure from his previous course, but that his forbearance is sought to be turned to his disadvantage, and objection is made to granting compensation by an act of Congress, on the ground that he ought to enforce his right under his patent against the officers of the United States using his discovery in the military, naval, and marine service, and against all persons violating the same. He therefore with great reluctance respectfully asks the government either to buy the patent or else to discontinue the use of ether.[10]

The petition was endorsed by 32 Senators and 116 Members of the House of Representatives, and others who said:

"The undersigned concur in recommending that the right to use Dr Morton's discovery, commonly called 'Practical Anaesthesia', be purchased for the public service or that the use thereof be discontinued, because the government is manifestly bound by its own patent, duly issued, to respect the said discovery as private property, and because *private property* ought not to be *taken for public use without just compensation*."[11]

Witte, the member for Pennsylvania, who had been staying next door to Morton, was on friendly terms with the President and offered to approach him on Morton's behalf. The President assured Witte that he would consider Morton's petition favourably, and referred it to the newly established Smithsonian Institution in Washington—named after the illegitimate son of the first Duke of Northumberland, a notable chemist and a Fellow of the Royal Society. Illegitimacy was almost a crime in England at that time and barred a man from inheriting, or from holding office in the

170

Church, a commission in the Armed Forces, or a seat in Parliament. "The best blood of England flows in my veins, on my father's side I am a Northumberland, on my mother's I am related to kings; but this avails me not." Leaving 105,000 gold sovereigns to found in America "an establishment for the increase and diffusion of knowledge among men", he said, "My name shall live in the memory of man when the titles of the Northumberlands and Percys are extinct and forgotten." Joseph Henry, the first head of this great institution and a famous physicist, was asked by the President to carry out one more impartial investigation into Morton's claim. His report, received by President Pierce in February 1855, once again stated that Morton had made the discovery.

Witte told Morton that the President was about to sign the Treasury order to compensate him for his patent, and that he had promised Witte an interview for March 15th, 1855. Eventually this was postponed until March 21st, and even then the President asked Witte to come back on March 23rd, when he promised he would have the documents ready. When Witte called upon the President on March 23rd the papers lay on his desk in front of him waiting for his signature, along with the report of the Smithsonian Institution, a petition from the Massachusetts General Hospital, Congressional Committee reports, and opinions from the Army and Navy Surgeons, all saying that Morton ought to be compensated. "It is earnestly hoped that our government, with a similar appreciation of this great acquisition to medical science, will stamp their sense of its importance by a substantial acknowledgement which will remunerate you in some measure for the toil and vexation attendant on your struggle for success,"[12] wrote the Surgeon of the Navy to Morton.

At last after all these years of struggle Morton was about to be given some recompense. The President started to sign. Suddenly he stopped. Something had caught his eye. "Other anaesthetic agents, this does not in any way militate against the merits of the original discovery . . ." said the testimonial from the Army Surgeon. "Other anaesthetic agents?" the President queried. What other agents were there then? What was the difference between them and ether? "There is a point," he said, "which is not yet exactly clear to my mind, as to whether the patent includes all anaesthetic substances for instance, chloroform; and for a little information on the subject, and to prevent any more doubt, I think it will be better to refer it to the Attorney-General, so that I can find exactly what the patent does cover."[13]

Witte protested that it was now nine years since Morton had made the discovery, that throughout this time the Government had been using his discovery without paying a cent for it, that during all these years it had been used to save the people of the United States their terrible sufferings, yet for all its value there had been no benefit to Morton—the discoverer. What possible justification could there be for a further interminable delay? The President hastened to assure Witte he would have the whole matter cleared up in no time at all and the papers signed within a very few days, and that he could assure Morton that the matter was as good as settled.

But while the Attorney-General went into the question, time passed, spring changed into summer, and summer into autumn. Morton left again for Etherton. There at least his careful plans, his scientific attention to detail, and his dogged persistence were beginning to bear fruit. His crops were splendid, his stock in fine fettle, and everything doing well. That autumn of 1855 Morton exhibited at the local show, and when the Agricultural Society of Norfolk County gave a dinner afterwards the list of prize-winners was read out: "First prize of twenty dollars for the most valuable and economical improvements in cultivation and management of a farm during the year—W. T. G. Morton; first prize of seventy dollars for the best dairy herd—W. T. G. Morton; best pair of farm horses—Morton; first prize for a Jersey cow—Morton's cow, Beauty; second prize —Morton's cow, Dairy Maid; butter, Ayrshires, Durhams, milking cows, heifers, swine, geese, turkeys, fowls—he got prizes for them all.

His farm was a showpiece; he was appointed Commissioner for the National Agricultural Society and asked to go as a delegate to the French Industrial Exhibition. Daniel Webster and others gave him introductions to important people in Europe, and Morton was looking forward to the trip. The Crimean War had started, and he planned to advise on the administration of ether to help the wounded there, but even here his opponents could not leave him alone and when they heard of his appointment they laid before the President of the Agricultural Society various scandalous matters, and Morton was forced to abandon his trip.

Their slanders were now so clever and insistent that even his own father-in-law was taken in, and Elizabeth Morton's mother wrote: "Your father is ashamed to leave the house. The newspapers are full of the scandal. How could William do such things?" Few like Morton's pastor ever bothered to investigate the matter fully for themselves, for he told Morton he had found the evidence was false, but otherwise kept the matter strictly to himself. Most were not so scrupulous, and soon the campaign of vilification unleashed by Jackson and his cronies boiled up into a rabid animosity against Morton, ending in an effigy of him being publicly burnt before his own house, in front of his terrified wife and young children.

When at first the news had got round that the President was going to compensate Morton for his patent, life had become easier for him, he had built up his home again, and his creditors had relaxed their pressure. The moneylenders rushed in to persuade him—with a good rate of interest to themselves—to pay off his friends at long last and to take up bills to tide him over until the Treasury note was paid. On the strength of his appointment to go to France he had leased his farm to friends for the small amount of 4500 dollars, and now took up a bill for a few thousand dollars here, a note of hand for 2000 dollars there, and so it went on until the loans mounted up and he was once more deeply committed.

Now when there seemed to be some doubt as to the President's real intention the moneylenders tried to call in their loans, and he was forced to pledge even his most cherished possessions; his library, his dental instruments, everything had to go to fend off his creditors and pay the expenses of his frequent visits to Washington. There he "haunted the anterooms of important personages from morning until long past noon", waiting for word from the President. Witte was exasperated at the long delay, and when at last he heard, wrote to the President: "The Hon. Attorney-General has this morning informed me that the government declines acting at this time, in the case of Dr Morton. . . ." Bitterly he complained how he had relied on "your declaration and absolute promise . . . never dreaming you would fail to do yourself, or to permit others to refuse doing an act, the justice and necessity of which you had more than once clearly admitted."[14]

President Pierce was a shifty character, one of the three about whom Whitman wrote: "History is to record those three Presidents . . . as so far our utmost warning and shame. Never were publicly displayed more deformed, mediocre, snivelling, unreliable, pulp-hearted men."[7] Witte, who had himself lent Morton money, concluded his letter to the President: "And yet, now, after the lapse of fourteen months, induced to come here often, and always at the sacrifice of my interests at home, I am told that there is nothing in the case—that the government refuses to acknowledge the slightest equity in the claim, but shielding behind legal quibbles and scientific technicalities, coolly and complacently pronounces its former assurances and promises of compensation and justice as nothing. . . .

"Well, sir, we must make submission, and we do submit in that feeling which injured helplessness makes to wrong and power."[15]

Morton was dismally disappointed. He suffered a second serious illness, but tried to secure an interview himself with the President. When a meeting was at last arranged by Senator Birkdale of Mississippi in the early part of May the President told Morton that he must secure a decision from the court as to the validity of his patent before any help could be given to him on the matter. It seemed most unfair. Morton had always been heavily criticized for having taken out a patent at all; now he was being told by the President himself that he should have taken steps to enforce it. Should he then for all these years have denied his discovery to the sick and the wounded? As Morton said in his petition: "Owing to the peculiar nature of his discovery, he had never wished to take legal steps for redress; that he had all along been led to suppose that the government would in the end act honestly, and for the good of humanity do, of its own free will, an act of justice, to which it was repugnant to human nature to compel it."[16]

173

The Government after all had itself been the first to infringe the patent, granted what is more by its own agency. Now President Pierce told Morton to start proceedings immediately against some surgeon in the Government service, assuring Morton that it was a mere formality. But in spite of all the President's assurances he was loath to take on the expense. For the sake of his wife and family, and his friends and creditors, he felt he should not add further to his responsibilities, for already he was inundated with writs, and attachments on his property were constantly being secured. Three writs alone amounting to some 10,000 dollars were served on him in one single day. He was advised by his pastor to go bankrupt, but Morton would not hear of evading his responsibilities like that. His position became worse. There was little money for food and none for clothes and other essentials. His family were almost in rags and were ridiculed and hooted at in the streets. Eventually his own possessions had gone, and he was forced to sell his children's piano and the pony that they loved so much.

A pawnbroker, Frederick T. Johnson, told what happened to one of Morton's most treasured possessions. He had a shop in the heart of Boston's shipping quarter, and his usual customers streamed in whenever times were bad to hand in little trinkets or bundles of clothing for money to buy food for their families. One day he was surprised to have an expensive case offered through his window. He watched as trembling hands took out a large gold medal set in an imposing laurel-wreath frame and lovingly wrapped in tissue-paper, with the inscription "Benefactor of Mankind". When Johnson questioned him closely whether he was entitled to the medal the thin, haggard man took from his pocket a creased and heavily worn piece of paper and showed him the citation. It was Morton himself. The pawnbroker named his price. Morton protested that it had cost much more, but Johnson insisted that he could give him only the bare value of the gold and Morton must take it or leave it. It was Morton's most treasured possession, but he was forced to accept, for he had a wife and family nearly starving and sentiment would not find them food.

Late in 1856 Amos Lawrence, one of the trustees of the Massachusetts General Hospital, got to hear of his plight and set about organizing a National Testimonial for Morton. The subscription list was opened in the following year, 1857, and appealed to all "Patrons of Science and the Friends of Humanity". The trustees voted one thousand dollars as a "memorial to his great services", and the Eye Infirmary gave two hundred. Lawrence himself gave one thousand, and all were asked to help. A group of New York doctors asked Nathan Rice to write Morton's story, and the book—*Trials of a Public Benefactor*—published in 1859, was dedicated as "one more attempt to procure justice". Written in a matter of months, it included a vast number of documents and letters and was largely Morton's own story. In fact, Rice claimed that Morton himself had added the title and much of the book without his permission, and later, in a fit of pique, Rice wrote an article[17] claiming that Wells was the real discoverer.

Morton meanwhile was uncertain about whether to take a case against the Government. Etherton had been pledged long ago and was about to be sold over his head when his lawyers sent him an urgent message: "Etherton can be saved, by instituting the suit against the government, as suggested by the President of the United States." Morton did not know what to do; should he take their advice and prosecute, or should he give it all up and go back to being an ordinary dentist or farmer? He felt he had a duty to all his friends who had so staunchly supported him through all the years and lent him money, and if there really was a possibility of winning a case against the Government and securing his patent he felt compelled to take it so that he could pay off his debts. Assured by the President himself that there would be no difficulty, persuaded by his lawyers and friends, and urged on by his own dogged persistence and determination to see justice prevail, he hastily scribbled on the bottom of the message "Do it", and handed it back to the messenger. Again he had joined fight, again he was to become embroiled in the expensive intricacies of the law, the world of politics, witnesses, statements, expensive and petty legal quibbles.

A naval doctor, Charles A. Davis, of the Marine Hospital near Boston, was selected to be named in the suit, and Morton's lawyers went to see him to explain that it was merely a test case. But the more Davis considered the matter, the more worried he became about its implications. He became even more worried when the Treasury Solicitor said he could expect no help from him, and refused him a Government lawyer. Davis was angry at being made the scapegoat for all the Government surgeons, and throughout the country doctors were outraged when they heard of Morton's action, declaring it utterly reprehensible to prosecute a doctor who had used Morton's discovery as part of his duty to save life.

Jackson too lost no time in turning the situation to his own advantage, and, further inflamed by him, it grew into a mass movement of condemnation against Morton, to oust him from the medical societies and to deprive him of his honorary doctorate of medicine. In Boston they were unsuccessful, thanks to the doctors of the hospital who remembered his great achievement and in his terrible dilemma regarded him with compassion. But in New York the American Medical Association pronounced him unworthy to be a member of their profession. But what was he to do, for he had been told by the President himself that it was a mere formality, a way of extracting a payment already promised him by the Government?

If it was a mere formality according to the President, Davis certainly did not take it that way, nor did Jackson, who had, it seemed, so kindly offered to help him. Putting their heads together to work out the best defence, they decided to prove that Long had used it some years before Morton and that therefore Morton was not the discoverer and the patent was invalid. By now it had also become apparent that, faced with having to pay for all the thousands of times it had been used to treat their wounded, the Government was no longer so ready to let him win. It was anyway nearly bankrupt then, and even had it been prompted by less cunning motives would have been forced to defend its position strenuously. This view was passed to the judiciary, at that time not unsympathetic to political influence.

Morton's lawyers proposed that he should prosecute a civil establishment too, and chose the New York Eye Infirmary, a private concern which had made his inhalers under licence for exporting abroad. This was an unwise move, as they were able to present a strong case for the defence, and Judge Shipman, who heard the case, decided against Morton and declared the patent invalid. A re-trial was applied for, and on December 1st, 1862, Shipman again pronounced judgement against Morton: "A discovery is not patentable. It is only where the explorer has gone beyond the domain of mere discovery and has laid hold of the new principle, force, or law, and connected it with some particular medium or mechanical contrivance. . . ."

But he went on: "Before dismissing the case, it may not be amiss to speak of the character of the discovery upon which the patent is founded. Its value . . . was proved. . . . Its discoverer is entitled to be classed among the greatest benefactors of mankind. But the beneficent and imposing character of the discovery cannot change the legal principles on which the law of patents is founded."[18]

Words, and more words, the most exalted tributes had been showered upon him, but of what help were they to poor Morton in his extreme condition? After sixteen years he was finished: tribunals, Congresses, Presidents, courts, he had appealed to them all for recompense and lost. Taunted into taking a case against the Government, promised hundreds of thousands of dollars, he had not been given a cent. "This," said Mrs Morton, "was perhaps the greatest sorrow of my husband's later years, a sorrow rendered all the more keen from the fact that other governments hastened to bestow upon him orders and decorations."[19] Utterly broken in health, deep in debt, and at last hopeless and disheartened, he returned home to Etherton. There everything he had cherished had been seized by the bailiffs, his beloved prize cows Beauty and Dairy Maid, his other animals, his famous geese, his marvellous new machines, his crops—everything had gone, his land stripped bare and sold to another. His starving wife and family were huddled together with hardly a stick of furniture, and but for the generosity of friends they would have had no roof over their heads. There at Etherton he faced stark poverty, unrelieved now by any hope of justice for his claim. He lived a pathetic and heart-rending existence, unbroken by any possibility of honour or reward for his great gift to mankind.

A friend of Edward Warren's, a traveller in farming implements, recounted how in the winter of 1863 he had gone out to West Needham. There he saw a thin, drawn, half-starved man, neatly dressed still, but in threadbare clothes, standing with a small handcart loaded with branches of wood, bargaining desperately with the baker's wife, trying to persuade her to let him have half a barrel of biscuit in exchange for the load of wood he had just gathered in the forest. Diffidently he begged for help for his wife and family who had had nothing to eat for days. This then was what Morton had been reduced to. This then was Dr Morton, Benefactor of Mankind, bestower of this greatest blessing, that gift from heaven. . . .

NOTES TO CHAPTER XVI

1. United States Congress, Statement supported by evidence of W. T. G. Morton, January 21st, 1853.
2. United States Congress, Committee Report.
3. United States Congress, Senate Report, 1853.
4. *Ibid.*
5. H. H. Young, *Long, the Discoverer of Anaesthesia.*
6. Nathan Rice, *Trials of a Public Benefactor.*
7. *Ibid.*
8. *Ibid.*
9. *Ibid.*
10. W. T. G. Morton, Petition to President, 1854.
11. *Ibid.*
12. Nathan Rice, *op. cit.*
13. *Ibid.*
14. *Ibid.*
15. *Ibid.*
16. W. T. G. Morton, *op. cit.*
17. Nathan Rice, "A Grain of Wheat from a Bushel of Chaff", in *Knickerbocker*, Vol. 53 (New York).
18. Federal Cases, Book 17, Morton's patent trial, December 1862.
19. *McClure's Magazine*, September 1896.

CHAPTER

XVII

I seems incredible that there is any doubt about who made the great discovery of anaesthesia. The Massachusetts General Hospital, where the first operation took place, the Army and Navy Surgeons, the Smithsonian Institution, and experts all over the world supported Morton. No fewer than six Congressional Committees confirmed him as the discoverer. "Morton alone proved the hypothesis," said Bigelow. "Without Morton there is no evidence that the world would have known ether until the present day." Its simple effects had been demonstrated for years, but until Morton had the courage and perception to make his great experiments no one had thought to take it further. For, as Bigelow pointed out: "Morton had a combination of qualities such as few other men in the community possessed. Fertile in expedients and singularly prompt in execution, he was earnest and persevering beyond conception. His determined persistence is remembered even at this interval of time, as having been a terror to his friends. Nobody denies that Morton recklessly and alone faced the then supposed dangers attending ether stupor. If all accredited scientific opinion had not been at fault, and in the case of any fatal result, he would infallibly have been convicted of manslaughter, with little possibility that anybody would have come forward to say: '*The responsibility is not his but mine.*'"[1]

"The great discovery, that for which the whole world is indebted," wrote G. P. Putnam, "was that the inhalation of ether could be employed with safety. . . . This, the only fact of real practical value, he proved, first by self-experiment, and he was the only man who ever proved it."[2]

In spite of all the abuse and vilification poured upon Morton he never retaliated. In spite of the strongest provocation he continued only to reiterate his own case. Wells said, "I have the utmost confidence in you as

178

a gentleman, and one who will ever aim to act your part well in accordance with the strictest honour and integrity. . . ."³ John J. May, a distinguished Bostonian, wrote of him:

I wish that you had known William Thomas Green Morton. I knew him well. I met him not infrequently in those years when the subject of anaesthesia engrossed his whole thought.

I like to bear him in mind as he was: a refined, courteous gentleman. Always neat in personal appearance, affable in manner, thoughtful of others' feelings and convenience, generous and warmly appreciative of any kindness and sign of good will offered him.

Though enterprising and ardent, and ever sanguine in business pursuits, in which he was remarkably methodical; and although often grieved and indignant at the gratuitous injuries and misrepresentations heaped upon him by unprincipled opponents, I do not remember that I ever heard from his lips an opprobrious epithet, or saw indications of an effort to retaliate upon his enemies.

Most of the other claimants deserved some credit, although they made their claim to success only after Morton had done the work. "It is probable," said Warren, "that Long performed three or four operations under anaesthesia and then abandoned his claims. . . . He is deserving of nothing but censure for not having appreciated the value of the agent." Had it been left to him humanity might still have been denied relief from pain. Wells too had great imagination, but he never managed to overcome the difficulties of administration, and nitrous oxide could not give the steady anaesthesia necessary for surgical operations. Jackson gave technical advice, but he had never administered ether or any other gas for an operation.

Davy, Faraday, Hickman, and Allen all did great work leading up to it, but as for some of the other contenders, "the large class of jump-up-behinders", as *The Lancet* called them, all they wanted was the honour and glory. Even Simpson himself claimed the discovery when he was asked to write an article for the *Encyclopaedia Britannica,* and he is usually given the credit in England. In actual fact Simpson did not use chloroform until more than a year after Morton's famous operation, and a year after he had seen ether successfully introduced into England. However, unlike the other claimants, Simpson was at least honourable at the last, and on his deathbed called for pen and ink and wrote to all those he had wronged in his lifetime to ask their forgiveness. Morton was dead by this time, but he wrote to Bigelow, for it was Dr Bigelow who had described Simpson as a man who wished to pose as a hero at Morton's cost. In his letter Simpson told Bigelow that he still believed chloroform to be a better anaesthetic, but that the credit should go to Morton, who by his discovery and its application had initiated "this new era in anaesthetics and surgery".⁴ Unfortunately history and opinion in England have not followed Simpson's lead, and Morton has never been given the honour he so richly deserves.

The most fascinating question, of course, is how Jackson came to have such success in his blatant attempt to steal Morton's discovery, and even more why he still gets credit in reference books today. Undoubtedly Morton was all too easily influenced, and his biggest mistake was taking Eddy's advice to let Jackson have a percentage of his patent. Once he had got a foot in the door Jackson secured an enormous advantage by being first to claim the discovery with his important friends in Europe. He then strengthened his position even further by having his paper printed as if it had the sanction of the American Academy. As Dana, Morton's lawyer, said: "Were it not for Dr Jackson's having stolen a march by announcing his discovery to all the scientific societies of Europe at once while Dr Morton was working here, and thus got votes passed and records made in his favour in Europe, before any facts were known . . . there would be no more question of Morton's claim than there is of Morse's, which Dr Jackson contested with equal zeal."

Jackson had a great reputation among his friends in Europe, and "the consequence is," said the *British and Foreign Medical Review* of July 1852, "that on the continent, at least, Dr Jackson has got the undeserved credit of having made a discovery which he at first ridiculed." The verdict of the European scientific societies was certainly crucial, for America was still a raw and unimportant country and its professions thought themselves vastly overshadowed. Daniel Drake when he was offered the Presidency of the American Medical Association in 1850 said: "I don't care to be brought into contact with the great physicians on the other side of the Atlantic, men of university education, whose advantages were so much greater than my own. I think too much of my country to place myself in so awkward a position."

Jackson's seniority, his position as a professor, and particularly his European education all played a part in Morton's failure, for few were prepared to question a professor's word against that of a mere toothpuller. People found it hard to believe that an uneducated dentist could make such a tremendous discovery, one which for centuries had eluded all the greatest scientific minds. Finally, there is no doubt that Jackson's malicious slanders prejudiced many people against Morton, until eventually his lies by their sheer insistent force began to take effect.

Not the least of all the factors which ruined Morton was Jackson's madness, for it was no normal mind—promises, declarations, honesty, they meant nothing to Jackson—a megalomaniac, dominated and obsessed by his overwhelming desire for power and importance. There was no manœuvre, no trick too low, no device too despicable, which he would not stoop to use to gain his object, the possession of Morton's discovery. His kind of madness was the more dangerous in that he appeared to be so

180

eminently reasonable, so charming and so placatory. This was a madness not easy to detect in its early years, and Morton was certainly no match for such evil genius.

Morton's desperate struggle for existence was momentarily ended when another battle began—the battle for freedom for the slaves. What had constantly overshadowed discussion of Morton's claim in Congress now sucked him into its vortex. As Rufus Choate—the eminent lawyer who advised Morton that his discovery was a proper subject for a patent—declared, Harriet Beecher Stowe's *Uncle Tom's Cabin* had betwixt night and morning created two million Abolitionists. Determined to stamp out slavery and to teach the South a lesson, the fire of discontent which had smouldered for years through the Union burst into flames when the South broke away to form the Confederate States. It was a desperate battle, and Morton was eventually drafted in as an unofficial anaesthetist for the thousands of wounded. Walt Whitman who served as an Army nurse with the Northern forces wrote a horrifying description of the scene:

"Outdoors, at the foot of a tree, within ten yards of the front of the house, I noticed a heap of amputated feet, legs, arms, hands, etc., a full load for a one horse cart. Several dead bodies lie near, each covered with its brown woollen blanket. The large mansion is quite crowded upstairs and down, everything impromptu, no system . . . all the wounds pretty bad, some frightful, the men in their old clothes, unclean and bloody. . . ."[5]

"Is this indeed humanity," he asks later, "these butchers' shambles? . . . There they lie . . . from 200 to 300 poor fellows—the groans and screams—the odour of blood, mixed with the fresh scent of the night, the grass, the trees—that slaughterhouse! Oh, well is it their mothers, their sisters cannot see them. . . . One man is shot by a shell, both in the arm and leg—both are amputated—there lie the rejected members. Some have their legs blown off—some bullets through the breast—some indescribably horrid wounds in the face or head, all mutilated, sickening, torn, gouged out—some in the abdomen—some mere boys. . . ."[6]

These were the patients Morton had come to save. John H. Brinton, Professor of Surgery at the Jefferson Medical College, Philadelphia, described meeting him there at the front. Brinton was at the headquarters of the Army of the Potomac in the early summer of 1864, when an aide entered and told General Grant that a civilian doctor—a stranger—wanted one of the horse-drawn ambulances to visit the field hospitals. The General refused immediately, saying that the ambulances were intended only for the wounded and in no circumstances could be taken for private use.

Brinton went out to tell the man who stood waiting in brown, travel-stained clothes outside the tent. It was Morton himself. When Brinton saw who it was he asked Morton to wait while he again approached Grant,

181

saying, "But, General, if you knew who that man is I think you would give him what he asks for."

Still the General emphatically refused, saying, "I will not divert an ambulance today for anyone. . . ." Brinton then told him that the stranger was Dr Morton, the discoverer of ether, and the General immediately agreed: "You are right, Doctor, he has done more for the soldier than anyone else, soldier or civilian, for he has taught you all to banish pain. Let him have the ambulance and anything else he wants."[7]

Afterwards, by order of the General Commanding, he was given the hospitalities of the headquarters, and allocated an ambulance, tent, mess, and servant. Morton gave his own view of the war in a letter written to a friend in May 1864:

> When there is any heavy firing heard, the ambulance corps, with its attendants, stationed nearest to the scene of action, starts for the wounded. The ambulances are halted near by, and the attendants go with stretchers and bring out the wounded. The rebels do not generally fire upon those wearing ambulance badges.
>
> Upon the arrival of a train of ambulances at a field hospital the wounds are hastily examined, and those who can bear the journey are sent at once to Fredericksburg. The nature of the operations to be performed on the others is then decided upon and noted upon a bit of paper pinned to the pillow or roll of blanket under each patient's head. When this had been done I prepared the patient for the knife, producing perfect anaesthesia in the average time of three minutes, and the operators followed, performing their operations with dexterous skill, while the dressers in their turn bound up the stumps.[8]

For the first time for many years Morton found solace in his work tending the wounded. For a while he forgot his own disappointments as he helped the endless procession of shattered bodies, working from dawn to dusk and even on into the night, anaesthetizing by the light of a lamp. "For myself," he said, "I am repaid for the anxiety and often wretchedness which I have experienced since I first discovered and introduced the anaesthetic qualities of sulphuric ether, by the consciousness that I have been the instrument of averting pain from thousands and thousands of maimed and lacerated heroes, who have calmly rested in a state of anaesthesia while undergoing surgical operations, which would otherwise have given them intense torture. They are worthy of a nation's gratitude —happy am I to have alleviated their sufferings."[9]

It was a bitter battle which divided the nation upon itself, and across the lines from Morton, separated only by the thin ranks of soldiers locked in the grips of that terrible internecine war, was Crawford Long, also ministering to the wounded, but on his side to the soldiers from the South —the Confederate armies. Long was now head of the military hospital at Athens, Georgia, which was overflowing with the constant stream of

182

wounded from General Lee's army. Pain was common to both sides, and Long used ether too in his operations on the wounded. As the Yankee armies swept south to engulf the Confederates, Long became more and more worried that his own home might be overrun by marauding soldiers, and, fearful about what might happen, he decided to send his eldest daughter to safety, along with some of their most valuable possessions. The carriage was loaded with all their silver and precious belongings and was just about to start when Long came running out of the house with a jar containing two gold watches and a roll of papers. Thrusting it into his daughter's hand, he said, "These are most important and under no circumstances must be lost; they are proofs of my discovery of anaesthesia. Promise me that when you reach your destination you will bury them in a secluded spot, but if overtaken by the raiders you may be frightened into giving them the jar if ordered to do so."

"I'll die before I do,"[10] cried the girl as she leapt into the carriage. When she got to safety she crept out at night with a friend into the woods, with the jar suspended on a cord tied round her waist. They dug a hole there, and she buried the jar as she had promised.

The war eventually ended in 1865, and the soldiers and the doctors who had tended them gradually drifted back to try to take up their old life again. But it had all changed. Long returned to his practice at Athens, but the old ways of ease and luxury were gone. His slaves had been freed, and all around him the plantations were desolate and the people ruined. He could not bear it and kept asking his family desperately over and over again, "What will become of us all?" He was getting old now, and the long rides out into the country to see his patients became more and more of a burden. His precious documents had been retrieved from their hiding-place, but no longer gave him any joy. He had thrust them away in an old battered green travelling trunk in an attic, and when he thought no one was looking he would steal up and sometimes spend hours going through the papers, his affidavits, the old receipt of Venables, and the other documents supporting his case. When they saw him go his family would say, "Father is attacked by the old fever," but they never dared mention the subject for fear of upsetting him. "My father," said his daughter, "was a man who bore disappointment and sorrow uncomplainingly, keeping them secret in his soul, lest others be made unhappy."[11] Long lived on for some thirteen years after the war, and strangely enough died one night of a heart-attack, just as he was administering ether to a woman in labour.

Morton did not last so long. He had regained his medal and a few meagre possessions, and returned again to West Needham. Still worried by his old nervous attacks, he could not wipe out the memory of his trials and disappointments. On July 6th, 1868, he received a registered letter from New York. Inside was a copy of an article by J. H. Abbott in the *Atlantic Monthly* resurrecting Jackson's claim and full of the old bitter libels. It was a long time since any such claim had been made, and his wife said, "The article agitated him to an extent I had never seen before."[12] It brought on another of his nervous spasms, but still he insisted that he must go at once to New York to refute the lies. Barely able to stand, with his hands trembling so much that he found great difficulty in holding anything, he spent some hours sorting out his papers—methodical to the last.

In New York he had an even more serious attack, and on July 11th they wired for his wife to come. She found him suffering, they thought, from some sort of rheumatism in one leg, but still hard at work with his lawyers preparing a suitable reply to the article. Ill though he was and against all advice, he continued working at great pressure. It was an extraordinarily hot summer, and the heat in New York was unbearable. On July 15th the house had been like an oven, with the windows and doors closed all day against the sun. One of his wife's relatives had lent them a carriage and that evening, to try to escape from the heat of the city, Morton suggested that they should drive to Washington Heights. They started off, but as they were going across Central Park his wife said:

He complained of feeling sleepy, but refused to give me the reins or to turn back. Just as we were leaving the park, without a word he sprang from the carriage, and for a few moments stood on the ground apparently in great distress. Seeing a crowd gathering about, I took from his pocket his watch, purse and also his two decorations and the gold medal. Quickly he lost consciousness, and I was obliged to call upon a policeman and a passing druggist, Dr Swann, who assisted me. We laid my husband on the grass, but he was past recovery. We sent at once for a double carriage, but it was an hour before one came. Then two policemen lifted him tenderly upon the seat, I being unable to do anything from the condition I was in: the horror of the situation had stunned me, finding myself alone with a dying husband, surrounded by strangers, in an open park at eleven o'clock at night.

We were driven at once to St Luke's Hospital, where my husband was taken in on the stretcher, and immediately the chief surgeon and house surgeons gathered about him. At a glance the chief surgeon recognised him, and said to me: "This is Dr Morton?"

I simply replied: "Yes."

After a moment's silence he turned to a group of house pupils and said: "Young gentlemen, you see lying before you a man who has done more for humanity and the relief of suffering than any man who has ever lived."

In the bitterness of the moment, I put my hand in my pocket, and, taking out the three medals, laid them beside my husband, saying: "Yes, and here is all the recompense he has ever received for it."[13]

So, on July 15th, 1868, at the early age of forty-eight, died William Thomas Green Morton—Benefactor of Mankind. Poverty, persecution,

184

suffering—he had borne them all. He had received little in his life but a few medals and honours, and there was little for his children. One son became a doctor and a psychiatrist, the second son served through the Zulu War and was awarded the Victoria Cross for bravery. Putnam in his letter had said: "Let us not decree a tablet on his tombstone, or ask of posterity to pay our debts with a monument,"[14] but he had gone unheeded. The grateful citizens of Boston erected a magnificent monument as his tombstone, with an inscription written by Dr Jacob Bigelow:

Wm. T. G. Morton
Inventor and Revealer of Anaesthetic Inhalation
By whom pain in surgery was averted and annulled
Before whom in all time surgery was agony
Since whom science has control of pain

Only Jackson lived on, still scanning all the reports, all the periodicals, for reference to the ether controversy or any mention of Morton's name. He spent hours writing unendingly, pamphlets, newspaper articles, reports to scientific bodies, and letters to his friends, correcting errors, and sending back proofs supposed to substantiate his own case. His hatred was unquenchable even five years after Morton's death, and he turned more and more to alcohol to find relief, until he became a chronic alcoholic.

In July 1873 in the middle of writing one more pamphlet, still continuing to vilify Morton's name, it is said he made his way in a drunken stupor towards Mount Auburn Cemetery. Stumbling over the grass towards Morton's monument, he gazed up at the inscription: "Revealer of Anaesthetic Inhalation—By whom pain in surgery was averted and annulled". As he stood there the memory of Morton must have seemed to shine more brightly, until the last thin thread of rationality was broken. Flaying about madly in the air with his arms, he screamed and screamed, his madness plain at last to all. Visitors tending near-by graves came running across to his convulsed body. Eventually the cemetery keeper and the police managed to hold down and bind the raging maniac. He was placed under restraint at the McLean Asylum and held there for the last seven years of his life, never apparently regaining his senses until he died on August 28th, 1880, at the age of seventy-five. Poor Jackson should be pitied too, for it was this madness that year after year had worn away all semblance of rationality, that vaunting ambition which eventually overreaches itself and leads to madness, a paranoia which had given birth to all his intrigues, his slanders, and his cunning plots to steal Morton's discovery.

For all the contenders, then, the fight was over. It is a strange sensation to stand today in beautiful Mount Auburn Cemetery, surrounded by so many of the cast in this sad story. Morton's memorial to the Benefactor of Mankind is set on the brow of the hill; Jackson's odd epitaph, "Thy God-like crime was to be kind, to render with thy precepts less, The Sum of human wretchedness", Bigelow, Bowditch, Oliver Wendell Holmes, Agassiz, Everett, Choate, Gould—they all lie there now. For the four contestants it might seem as if a curse had been laid upon them, for they all died unhappily: Wells became addicted to chloroform and killed himself; Morton died heartbroken and penniless; Long became an embittered old man; Jackson's madness deepened until he was incarcerated in a lunatic asylum.

After their death memorials sprang up everywhere: Connecticut erected a monument to Wells in Bushnell Park, Hartford, and in 1937 a carved pew in the chapel of Trinity College there. Georgia erected a statue to Long in the National Capitol. Massachusetts added Morton's name to the roll of honour, second in the list of fifty-two of its greatest sons, his name inscribed at the head of one of the pillars in Boston State House; there is the monument over his grave, another in the Boston Public Garden, and the Ether Dome is itself preserved in the Massachusetts General Hospital to his memory and to all those who took part in the momentous operation on October 16th, 1846.

In the building adjoining the Royal College of Surgeons in Lincoln's Inn Fields hangs an engraving of the members of the Council of the College in 1884, all posed in solemn splendour, among them Lord Lister, and Cadge, who had assisted Liston in the first operation performed with ether in England, now promoted to seniority. At the bottom, almost in the margin, added as an afterthought—twenty years after his death and forty years after his great discovery—is a tiny portrait of Morton, with the inscription "Anaesthesia, U.S.A." It seems to indicate an informal election to Fellowship of the College, but even in this high place of honour Morton does not entirely win the day, for instead of W. Morton, it reads C. (as if for Charles) Morton. Even here, Professor Charles Jackson seems still to claim half the honour.

NOTES TO CHAPTER XVII

1. H. J. Bigelow, *History of the Discovery of Modern Anaesthesia*, American Journal of Medical Science, 1876, 141.
2. Nathan Rice, *Trials of a Public Benefactor*.
3. *Ibid.*
4. James Simpson, Letter to Bigelow, *Boston Gynaecological Journal*, May 1870.
5. *Specimen Days*: "Down at the Front".
6. *Specimen Days*: "A Night Battle".
7. Quoted by Mrs Morton in *McClure's Magazine*, September 1896.
8. *Ibid.*
9. *McClure's Magazine*, September 1896.
10. Frances Long Taylor, *Crawford W. Long and the Discovery of Ether Anaesthesia*.
11. *Ibid.*
12. *McClure's Magazine*, September 1896.
13. *Ibid.*
14. Nathan Rice, *op. cit.*

BIBLIOGRAPHY

ABBOT, J. H.: "Principles Recognized by Scientific Men Applied to the Ether Controversy", *Littell's Living Age*, 1848, No. 2148, 17, pp. 565–569.
————: "The Discovery of Etherization", *Atlantic Monthly*, November 1896, 78, pp. 679–686.
Académie des Sciences: *Compte rendu*, Tom. 24, 1847, Paris.
————: *Compte rendu des séances de l'académie des sciences*, I, semestre, 1850, Paris.
Académie Royale de Médecine: Bulletin XII, année II, 1846–47, Paris.
Anaesthetic and Analgesia: A Visit to the Birthplace of William Morton, 1932, No. 3, p. 45.
Annals of Medical History, 1925, VII, pp. 267–296.
————: November 3rd, 1931.
ARCHER, WILLIAM H.: "Chronological History of Horace Wells, Discoverer of Anaesthesia", *Bulletin of the History of Medicine*, 1939, 14, pp. 71–77.
————: "Life and Letters of Horace Wells", *Journal of the American College of Dentists*, 1944, 11, 83; 1945, 12, 85.
ARNOLD, HOWARD PAYSON: *Memoirs of Jonathan Mason Warren, M.D.*, Boston, 1886.
AYER, W.: *Account of an Eye-Witness of the First Public Demonstration of Ether-Anaesthesia, etc.*
BARKERS, S. W.: "An Interview with William Morton", *Harper's Magazine*, 1865, No. 31, pp. 453–460.
BEECHER, H. K.: "The First Anaesthesia Records", *Surg. Gynaec. Obstet.*, 1940, 71, pp. 689–693.
BEMIS, C. V.: "Personal Recollections of the Introduction of Anaesthesia", *Boston Medical and Surgical Journal*, 1891, Vol. 86, No. 1.
BIGELOW, HENRY JACOB, M.D.: "A History of the Discovery of Modern Anaesthesia", *American Journal of Medical Science*, 1876, 141, pp. 164–184.
————: "Insensibility during Surgical Operations Produced by Inhalation", *Boston Medical and Surgical Journal*, November 18th, 1846, pp. 309–317.
————: *Surgical Anaesthesia*, Boston, 1900.
BIGELOW, JOHN: *The Mystery of Sleep*, New York, 1877.
BOLAND, F. K.: "Crawford W. Long", *Bulletin Hist. Med.*, 1942, 12, pp. 191–225.
Boston Daily Advertiser, March 19th, 1870.

187

Boston Medical and Surgical Journal: Articles about the introduction of ether anaesthesia, November 18th and December 9th, 1846.

————: "Debate in Senate", Supplement to *Journal*, 1852.

BOWDITCH, NATHANIEL I.: *A History of the Massachusetts General Hospital, 1810–1851*, Boston, 1851.

————: *The Ether Controversy, Vindication of Morton in Reply to Jackson's Claims after Report of Trustees of the Massachusetts General Hospital*, Boston, 1848.

CLENDENING, LOGAN: *Source Book of Medical History*, New York, 1942.

COCK, F. W.: "The First Major Operation Under Ether in England", *American Journal of Surgery*, 1915, 29; (Anaesthesia Supplement), 98.

COLLYER, R. H.: "History of the Anaesthetic Discovery", *The Lancet*, 1917.

COLTON, G. Q.: *A True History of the Discovery of Anaesthesia*, New York, 1896.

————: *Anaesthesia, Who Made and Developed This Great Discovery?* New York, 1886.

Committee of Citizens of Boston, *Historical Memorandum*, 1871.

COTTING, BENJAMIN EDDY: "A Bit of Professional Reminiscence, Etherwise and Otherwise", *Boston Medical and Surgical Journal*, 1897, 136, I.

CRAWFORD, M. C.: *Old Boston Days and Ways*, Boston, 1924.

————: *Romantic Days in the Early Republic*, Boston, 1912.

DANA, R. H.: "Report of the Trustees of the Massachusetts General Hospital", *Littell's Living Age*, March 1848.

DAVY, HUMPHRY: *Researches, Chiefly Concerning Nitrous Oxide*, London, 1800.

DUNCUM, BARBARA: *The Development of Inhalation Anaesthesia*, London, 1947.

EMERSON, RALPH WALDO: *A History of the Gift of Painless Surgery*, Boston, 1896.

————: "The Discovery of Etherization", *Atlantic Monthly*, November 1896, 78, pp. 679–686.

ESDAILE, JAMES: *Mesmerism in India, and Its Practical Application in Surgery and Medicine*, London, 1846.

Federal Cases, Book 17, Morton's Patent Trial, December 1862.

FLAGG, J. F. B.: *Ether and Chloroform, Their Employment in Surgery, Dentistry and Midwifery*, Philadelphia, 1851.

Full Exposure of C. T. Jackson's Conduct, leading to the Discharge from the Government Service, and Justice to Messrs Foster and Whitney, U.S. Geologists.

FULTON, JOHN F., and STANTON, MADELINE: *An Annotated Catalogue of Books, etc., on the Early History of Surgical Anaesthesia*, New York, 1946.

GALLOUPE, ISAAC F.: "Personal Recollections of the First Use of Anaesthetics", *Boston Medical and Surgical Journal*, Vol. 86, No. 1, 1891.

————: "Reminiscences of the Harvard Medical School in the Year 1846", *Boston Medical and Surgical Journal*, 131, 426, 1894.

GAY, MARTIN: *A Statement of the Claims of Dr Charles T. Jackson, M.D., etc.*, Boston, 1847.

Georgia University: *Special Series Addresses*, I, No. 14, 1927, pp. 1–12.

GOLDSMITH, MARGARET: *Franz Anton Mesmer*, London, 1934.

GRANDY, LUTHER B.: *A Contribution to the History of the Discovery of Modern Surgical Anaesthesia*, Richmond, 1893.

————: "The Discovery of Anaesthesia", *New York Medical Journal*, July 20th, 1896.

HALE, SARAH J.: *Godey's Lady's Book*, 1853, 46, pp. 205–212.

Hartford Courant, Dec. 10th, 1844.

HAYWARD, G.: *Some Account of the First Use of Sulphuric Ether by Inhalation in Surgical Practice*, Boston, 1847.

188

HODGES, RICHARD M.: *A Narrative of Events Connected with the Introduction of Sulphuric Ether into Surgical Use,* Boston, 1891.

HOLMES, OLIVER WENDELL: "Anaesthesia", *Century Magazine,* 1893.

Illustrated London News, Jan. 9th, 1847, 10, 30.

Institut de France, Académie des Sciences: *Rapports de prix, Programme des Concours,* 1841–1855.

JACKSON, CHARLES T.: *A Manual of Etherization,* Boston, 1861.

JACKSON, J. B. S.: "Review of Dr Martin Gay's Statement of Dr Charles T. Jackson's Claims", *Boston Medical and Surgical Journal,* June 30th, 1847, 36, 429.

JACOBS, J.: *Dr Crawford W. Long,* Atlanta, 1919.

KENDALL, AMOS: *Morse's Patent, Full Exposure of Dr Charles T. Jackson's Pretensions to the Invention of the American Electromagnetic Telegraph,* Washington, 1852.

KEYS, T. E.: *History of Surgical Anaesthesia,* New York, 1945.

Littell's Living Age: "Report of the Trustees of the Massachusetts General Hospital", 1848, No. 201, 16, 556.

————: "Memorial by the Massachusetts General Hospital to the Senate and House of Representatives", 1848, No. 201, 16, 563.

London People's Journal: Article about the introduction of ether in surgical practice, January 9th, 1847.

LONG, CRAWFORD W.: "An Account of the First Use of Sulphuric Ether by Inhalation as an Anaesthetic in Surgical Operations", *Southern Medical and Surgical Journal,* 5 (new series), 705, 1849.

LORD, J. L., and LORD, H. C.: "A Defence of Dr Charles T. Jackson's Claims to the Discovery of Etherization", *Littell's Living Age,* 1848, 17, 491.

————: *Memorial addressed to the Trustees of the Massachusetts General Hospital in behalf of Charles T. Jackson, M.D.,* Boston, 1849.

MACMANUS, JAMES: *Notes on the History of Anaesthesia,* Hartford, 1894.

————: *The Wells Memorial Celebration, Notes on the History of Anaesthesia,* Hartford, 1901.

Massachusetts General Hospital: *Semi-Centennial of Anaesthesia, 1846–1896,* Boston, 1897.

————: *Bylaws, Annual Report, 1846–47,* Boston, 1847.

MAUPASSANT, GUY DE: *L'Endormeuse.*

MILLER, ALBERT H.: "The Origin of the Word Anaesthesia", *Boston Medical and Surgical Journal,* 1927, 197, pp. 1218–22.

————: "Two Notable Controversies over the Invention of the Electric Telegraph and the Discovery of Surgical Anaesthesia", *Annals of Medical History,* New York, March 1934.

MILLER, ALBERT H.: *Thomas Beddoes, Pioneer in Inhalation Therapy,* New York, 1932.

MILLER, WILLIAM: *A New History of the United States,* New York, 1958.

MORTON, ELIZABETH WHITMAN: "The Discovery of Anaesthesia", *McClure's Magazine,* September 1896.

MORTON, W. J.: *Memoranda relating to the Discovery of Surgical Anaesthesia, Postgraduate,* 1905.

MORTON, W. T. G.: *Appeal to the Patrons of Science, etc.,* 1856.

————: *Circular on Letheon,* 1847.

————: *Memoir to the Academy of Arts and Sciences of Paris,* 1847.

————: *On the Physiological Effects of Sulphuric Ether,* 1850.

————: *Pain and Anaesthesia,* Washington, 1863.

————: *Proceedings in Behalf of the Morton Testimonial,* Boston, 1861.

————: "A Speech", *Cincinnati Gazette,* December 28th, 1866.

————: *Testimonial* (Report to Congress including petition, letters, etc.) 38th Congress, 1864.

————: *The Use of Ether as an Anaesthetic at the Battles of the Civil War*, Chicago, 1904.

————: and JACKSON, C. T., U.S. Patent No. 4848, November 12th, 1846.

New York: Appeal to public by members of the medical profession in New York, 1858.

New York Daily Tribunal: January 24th, 25th, and 26th, 1848.

New York Evening Post: January 17th and 27th, 1848; also May 26th and 29th and June 30th, 1873.

New York Herald: January 23rd and 25th, 1848.

Old Home Day, to erect memorial, 1920.

OSLER, SIR WILLIAM: "The First Printed Documents relating to Modern Surgical Anaesthesia", *Annals of Medical History*, 1910, I, pp. 329–332.

OTIS, SIDNEY: Letter from Mrs Edward Whitman about the marriage of her daughter with Dr Morton.

PARKER, GEORGE: "The Discovery of the Anaesthesia Powers of Nitrous Oxide", *The Lancet*, January 7th, 1928.

PEREIRA, JONATHAN: *Elements of Materia Medica*, London, 1839.

POORE, BENJAMIN PORLEY: *Historical Materials for the Biography of W. T. G. Morton, M.D., Discoverer of Etherization; with an account of Anaesthesia*, Washington, 1856.

Practitioner, The: Heroes of Medicine, "Robert Liston", 10 (new series), 546, 1899.

RAEDER, O. M.: *America in the Forties*, Minnesota, 1929.

RICE, NATHAN P.: *Trials of a Public Benefactor*, New York, 1859.

————: "A Grain of Wheat from a Bushel of Chaff", *The Knickerbocker*, 1859, 53, pp. 133–138.

SIMPSON, SIR JAMES: Letter to Bigelow, *Boston Gynaecological Journal*, May 1870.

————: *Landmarks in the Struggle between Science and Religion*.

SMILIE, E. R.: *An Address . . . on the History of the Original Application of Anaesthetic Agents, May 17th, 1848*, Boston, 1848.

SMITH, TRUMAN: *An Examination of the Question of Anaesthesia, etc.* New York, 1858.

————: *An Inquiry into the Origin of Modern Anaesthesia*, Hartford, 1867, including a "Life of Horace Wells", by P. W. Ellsworth.

STANLEY, EDWARD and EVANS, ALEXANDER: *Report to the House of Representatives of the United States, Vindicating the Rights of Charles T. Jackson to the Discovery of the Anaesthetic Effect of Ether Vapour*, Boston, 1852.

STOCK, JOHN E.: *Memoirs of the Life of Thomas Beddoes, M.D.*, London, 1811.

TAYLOR, FRANCES LONG: *Crawford W. Long and the Discovery of Ether Anaesthesia*, New York, 1927.

United States Congress: *Congress Report*, 1849.

————: *Minority Report*, 1849.

————: *Report on the Ether Discovery*, 1852.

————: House of Representatives: two *Reports* in 1852, on the memorial of W. T. G. Morton.

————: *Minority Reports* on Dr Morton, 1852.

————: *Statement* for Jackson, 1852.

————: *Statement supported by Evidence of W. T. G. Morton, M.D., on his Claim submitted to the Select Committee appointed by the Senate of the United States*, January 21st, 1853.

————: *Senate Report*, 1853.

————: *Proceedings*, 1854.

————: *Senate Report*, 1863.

————: *Petition for Dr Morton*, 1863.

————: *Testimonial Report to Congress*, including petition, letters, etc., to 38th Congress, 1864.

VIETS, HENRY R.: *Brief History of Medicine in Massachusetts*, Boston and New York, 1930.

WARREN, EDWARD: *Some Account of Letheon*, Boston, 1847.

WARREN, J. COLLINS: "Insensibility during Surgical Operations produced by Inhalation", *Boston Medical and Surgical Journal*, 35, No. 16, 1846.

————: *The Influence of Anaesthesia on the Surgery of the Nineteenth Century*, Boston, 1897.

WELCH, WILLIAM H.: *A Consideration of the Introduction of Surgical Anaesthesia*, Boston, 1908.

WELLS, HORACE: *A History of the Discovery of the Application of Nitrous Oxide Gas, etc.*, Hartford, 1847.

————: Letter to the Editor, *Boston Medical and Surgical Journal*, 36, 421, 1847.

————: Letter to the Editor, *Hartford Courant*, December 7th, 1846.

Horace Wells Centenary Committee of the American Dental Association 1948: *Horace Wells, Dentist, Father of Surgical Anaesthesia*.

Discovery by the late Dr Horace Wells (Hartford case, 1850).

Dr Wells, the Discoverer of Anaesthesia, New York, 1860.

WOODWORTH, J. B. L.: Article on Chas. T. Jackson, including complete bibliography of his writings, *American Geologist*, 1897, 20, 70, etc.

YOUNG, H. H.: "Long, the Discoverer of Anaesthesia, a Presentation of his Original Documents, John Hopkins Hospital Bulletin, 8, 174, 1897.

INDEX

ABBOTT, GILBERT, subject of first public demonstration of ether anaesthesia, 70–71, 73–75, 78

Abbott, J. H., 183

Agassiz, Professor Louis, 126, 132

Agricultural Society of Norfolk County, 172

American Academy of Arts and Sciences, 93, 123–125, 151, 157, 180

American Civil War, Morton an unofficial anaesthetist in, 181–183

American Dental Association, 100

American Medical Association, 175, 180

American Society of Dental Surgeons, 20, 23

'Anaesthesia', choice of name, 111–112

Angell, Dr G. M., 89–90

Aphrodite, 30

Apollonia, St, 29

Athens (Georgia), 167, 182–183

Atlantic Monthly, 183

BACON, FRANCIS, 106

Bacon, R. H., 153

Badger, Senator, 162

Bailly (Troyes barber-surgeon), 30

Baltimore College of Dental Surgery, 20–21

Baltimore Sun, 160

Beaumont, Élie de, 49, 150, 152, 153; Jackson writes to, 110, 113, 117; reads out Jackson's claim to French Academy, 116, 118, 119, 123; Jackson's book dedicated to, 158

Beaumont, William, and gastric experiments, 49–59, 107, 109, 117, 142

Beddoes, Dr Thomas, 36, 38

Benedict, St, 30

Benton, Senator, 17

Bigelow, Henry J., 78, 90, 91, 92, 93, 122, 124, 137, 143, 178; supports Morton, 69–70, 73, 105, 147; at his first public ether demonstration, 73; his paper on the new discovery, 93, 106, 107, 108, 113, 117; on free availability of ether, 102; and Jackson's claim, 108, 109; Simpson's letter to, 179

Bigelow, Dr Jacob, 29, 69, 73, 94, 117; his epitaph on Morton, 185

Birkdale, Senator, 173

Blasius, the Blessed, 29

Boott, Dr Francis, 94, 159

Borland, Senator, 161, 167

Boston, *passim*; Morton in partnership with Wells in, 21–22; his struggle alone in, 22–24, 27 *et seq.*; Harvard Medical School, 27, 28–29; Beacon Hill (Jackson's home), 28, 60; citizens' testimonial to Morton, 146–147; Morton's monument in Mount Auburn Cemetery, 185, 186

LAFAYETTE, MARQUIS DE, 31

Lagenbeck (Hanoverian Army chief surgeon), 67

Lancet, The, 97, 99, 101, 103, 107, 179

Laughing gas (nitrous oxide), 38–44; Davy's preparation of, 36; inhalation made illegal, 38; exploited by travelling showmen, 39–40; Wells' use of in dentistry, 41–43; failure of demonstration, 43–44, 69, 114; improved technique of, in dentistry, 138, 158

Lavoisier, Antoine, 32

Lawrence, Amos, 174

Leavitt (apprentice), 57, 60

Leicester Academy, 17

'Letheon' suggested as name for anaesthetics, 111, 112

Lincoln, Abraham, 99

Lister, Lord, 103

Liston, Robert, 67, 68; first operation with ether in England, 94–97, 99–100

Littell's Living Age, 141

Long, Crawford Williamson: experiments with ether, 46–49, 167; claim to discovery of anaesthesia, 167–168, 179, 183; during Civil War, 182–183; memorial to, 186

Louis XVI, 32

Lully, Raymond, 38

McCORMICK, CYRUS HALL, 99

Magendie, François, 104

Magnetism, 31–33

Mallory, Senator, 163

'Man with the window in his stomach', 49–50

Mandragora, as pain-killer, 30

Manual of Etherization (Jackson), 158–159

Marcou, Jules, 154

Marcy, Dr, 165, 168

Marie Antoinette, 31

Massachusetts General Hospital, 33, 42, 124, 149, 159, 171, 178; Bigelow visiting surgeon to, 70; Morton administers ether in operation at, 70, 72–76, 78–79; Ether Dome, 73, 186;

operation on Alice Mohan at, 88–92; insists on Morton naming preparation, 91–92; Committee of Inquiry into claims, 136–139, 147, 155; doctors' petition to Congress, 143, 147

Massachusetts Mechanical Asociation, 22

Massachusetts Medical College, 28

Massachusetts Medical Society, 128; forbids 'secret remedies', 83–84; opposes Morton's use of inhaler for profit, 88, 90–91; impressed by Jackson's repudiation of patent, 131–132, 133

Maupassant, Guy de, on use of ether for migraine, 38

May, John J., 179

Medical and Surgical Journal (Boston), 79

Medical Examiner (Philadelphia), 104

Medical Journal (Orleans), 104

Medical Times, 104

Memoir on Sulphuric Ether (Morton), 56, 71, 138, 141, 151

Mesmer, Anton, and theory of animal magnetism, 31–33

Metcalf (Boston druggist), 53, 59, 138

Mexican War: Morton's inhaler rejected for use in, 121–122; inhaler used without compensation in, 131, 143

Mitchell, Dr Lantham, 38

Mohan, Alice, major painless surgery on, 88–92, 107

Montgomery, Dr, 105

Montyon Prize, 152–154

Morse, Samuel, 99; his invention of telegraph challenged by Jackson, 50–52, 107, 117

Morton, Elizabeth (wife), 25–28, 34, 55–56, 61–62, 72, 73, 74–75, 77, 169, 184

Morton, James (father): buys farm near Charlton, 14; insists on education for his children, 15; buys village store, 16, 17; other business ventures, 17; loses money, 17–18

197

Morton, Robert (ancestor), 13

Morton, William: birth and ancestry, 13–15; early schooldays, 15–16; work on family farm, 15; religious education, 16; ambition to learn medicine, 16; at Oxford Academy, 16; health ruined by unjust punishment, 16; at Northfield and Leicester Academies, 17; forced to leave school on father's failure, 18; clerk in Boston printing office, 18; failure of mercantile career, 18; sets up dental practice, 21; partner with Wells, 21–22; struggles on in Boston, 22, 27; buys Keep's trade secrets, 23; makes false teeth, 23–24, 29; meets future wife in Farmington, 25–26; courtship and marriage, 26–27; studies at Harvard Medical School, 27–29; boards and studies with Jackson, 28, 34, 49, 140; studies pain-killers, 30, 31–33, 53; uses ether on dental patient, 34; realizes value as pain-killer, 34; experiments on birds and animals, 35, 44, 56–57; failure of Wells' nitrous oxide demonstration, 43–44; leaves Jackson's house after quarrel, 52; reads of ether inhalation, 53; warned of dangers, 53; gives up practice to concentrate on experiment, 53–54, 56 *et seq.*; builds house at West Needham, 55; tries in vain to persuade someone to inhale ether, 58; tries it on himself, 58, 61–62; puzzled over varying results, 58–59; procures gasbag from Jackson, 59–60, 140; discovers pure ether to be remedy, 60–65, 140; his first dental operation with it, 62; exploits painless extractions, 62–65; Jackson's scepticism over, 63–64; difficulties in perfecting method, 64–65, 70, 77–78; realizes possibility of use in surgery, 65, 69; resumes experiments, 69; rebuffs from doctors, 69; administers ether at Massachusetts General Hospital, 70, 72–76, 77–79;

worry over apparatus, 71–72; triumph, 76; publicizes success, 78–81; tries to appoint Wells as agent, 79–80, 87; offers licences to doctors and dentists, 80–81; efforts to secure patent, 81–85, 87; surprised at Jackson's claim for compensation, 81–82; agrees to pay 500 dollars, 82, 83; and Jackson's claim to 10 per cent of profits, 84–85; agrees to this, 85; criticized for using invention for profit, 88, 90–91; operation on Alice Mohan, 88–92, 107; forced to disclose contents of preparation, 91–92; Warren's eulogy of, 93; granted patent, 99; applies for patents abroad, 99; partnership with Keep, 100; ethics of licensing use, 100–103; condemned by doctors and dentists, 103–106, 114; perfects method, 106, 112; amazed at Jackson's claims, 108–109; names process 'anaesthesia', 111–112; grandiose plans, 112–113; increasing claims of Jackson, 114–115; astounded by Jackson's claim to French Academy, 115–119; deceived by promise to 'put things right', 119–120, 123, 125, 131; Keep ends partnership, 121; increasing opposition, 121; offers inhalers to Army in Mexican War, 121–122; Jackson's vicious campaign against, 122–123, 127, 129–130, 132, 148–149; tricked by Jackson's false report of French Academy proceedings, 124–125; continues to seek settlement, 125–128; reputation undermined, 129–130; collapse of plans after patent nullified, 131–133; strange plots against, 133–136; patients alienated, 134–136; financial ruin, 136, 141; Committee of Inquiry, 136–139; assembles facts in *Memoir*, 138; applies for Government recognition of discovery, 142–143, 147–151; destitution and broken health, 146, 163–164; fund and testimonial, 146–147;